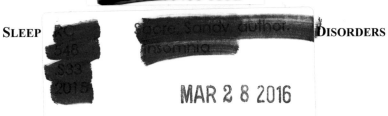
INSOMNIA

A SELF HELP HANDBOOK

SLEEP - PHYSIOLOGY, FUNCTIONS, DREAMING AND DISORDERS

Additional books in this series can be found on Nova's website under the Series tab.

Additional e-books in this series can be found on Nova's website under the e-book tab.

INSOMNIA

A SELF HELP HANDBOOK

SANDY SACRE, PH.D.

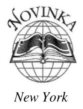

New York

NOTICE TO THE READER

The Publisher has taken reasonable care in the preparation of this book, but makes no expressed or implied warranty of any kind and assumes no responsibility for any errors or omissions. No liability is assumed for incidental or consequential damages in connection with or arising out of information contained in this book. The Publisher shall not be liable for any special, consequential, or exemplary damages resulting, in whole or in part, from the readers' use of, or reliance upon, this material. Any parts of this book based on government reports are so indicated and copyright is claimed for those parts to the extent applicable to compilations of such works.

Independent verification should be sought for any data, advice or recommendations contained in this book. In addition, no responsibility is assumed by the publisher for any injury and/or damage to persons or property arising from any methods, products, instructions, ideas or otherwise contained in this publication.

This publication is designed to provide accurate and authoritative information with regard to the subject matter covered herein. It is sold with the clear understanding that the Publisher is not engaged in rendering legal or any other professional services. If legal or any other expert assistance is required, the services of a competent person should be sought. FROM A DECLARATION OF PARTICIPANTS JOINTLY ADOPTED BY A COMMITTEE OF THE AMERICAN BAR ASSOCIATION AND A COMMITTEE OF PUBLISHERS.

Additional color graphics may be available in the e-book version of this book.

LIBRARY OF CONGRESS CATALOGING-IN-PUBLICATION DATA

ISBN: 978-1-63321-919-9

Library of Congress Control Number: 2014950568

Published by Nova Science Publishers, Inc. † New York

And if tonight my soul may find her peace in sleep, and sink in good oblivion, and in the morning wake like a new-opened flower then I have been dipped again in God, and new-created.

- D.H. Lawrence

CONTENTS

PREFACE

Insomnia is one of the most common reasons why people visit their physicians or general practitioners. It affects most people at some point in their lives. Yet, the treatments prescribed are often sedative medications that are only useful in the short-term, often have side effects and can lead to dependence. This handbook will show how insomnia sufferers can simply and effectively resolve their own sleep difficulties by using some evidence based, self-help techniques. The Cognitive Behavioral Therapy strategies that are taught in this handbook can be used at home and have been shown by sleep research to be the most effective and cost-effective therapies available for the treatment of insomnia.

I have worked as a health professional and educator for over 35 years and during this time have encountered many clients with insomnia. In some of my research and clinical work, I have specialized in Cognitive Behavioral Therapy for insomnia. My research has shown that safe and effective techniques for managing insomnia can be mastered by individuals, if they are given accurate information and easy to follow instructions and encouragement to persevere with using these approaches long-term. This handbook provides this information and these instructions so that even long-term insomnia sufferers can learn to successfully manage their sleep problems and prevent insomnia from recurring in the future.

When I began looking for books that I might be able to recommend to my insomnia clients, I could not find a book that was easy to digest and jargon-free and also based on what the current research evidence was showing. Many books on the market were highly technical and therefore hardly useful to insomnia sufferers looking for clear, readily understandable information and straightforward strategies. Some of the books that were aimed at insomnia sufferers went into a lot of detail about technical aspects of sleep and insomnia that were really not that important to people who just want to address the problem. While I believe that understanding the problem is important, I think it is only necessary to a certain degree. I'll provide you with some basic information about the biology of sleep and some insights into interesting sleep research but I won't burden you with too much of that in this handbook.

Another thing I found when I was looking around at what was available was that many books were aimed at clinicians. The irony here is that many clinicians have relatively little time with their clients and are therefore unable to deliver the kind of therapy required for insomnia. The good news is this: With little or no support from clinicians, most people with insomnia can help themselves! You just need some guidance and encouragement to persevere with techniques and strategies that can all be taught in a handbook like this one.

So the journey began. I decided to develop a handbook that was less of a textbook and more of a user-friendly handbook that explains what insomnia is and how it is caused and perpetuated and then demonstrates what sufferers can do to manage and eliminate the problem. Unless there are complicating factors, people with insomnia can work through this handbook themselves with minimal (or possibly no) assistance from their clinician. Even if you have other physical or psychological conditions as well, you may still be able to work on your insomnia yourself, alongside the accompanying treatment you are receiving for those other conditions from a health professional. As such, the uses of this handbook are broad, flexible and practical.

ACKNOWLEDGMENTS

I would like to thank all of my patients and research participants for all that they have taught me about the lived experience of insomnia. You have helped me to understand what it is like to endure the consequences of sleep loss and also to examine what helps and what doesn't. I know that your contribution to my knowledge about insomnia has helped me greatly in designing this handbook to be a practical guide to others in the same situation.

Many thanks to my husband and son, who have long endured my own late nights and busy days while I have been at work writing this handbook – thank you both for your patience and love.

Thanks to my mother who first taught me the importance of good sleep hygiene and regular bedtimes, habits that are critical to good health and childhood learning. I haven't always adhered to best practice in this regard, but I think my mother gave me a good foundation.

Thank you to my father who instilled in me a great wonder about all things mysterious, which led to my interest in the largely unknown scientific frontier of sleep psychology. He has also been a great support throughout my many years of clinical work, learning and research. This book is dedicated to you, Dad.

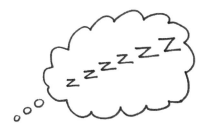

INTRODUCTION

Come, cuddle your head on my shoulder, dear, your head like the golden-rod, and we will go sailing away from here to the beautiful land of Nod.

- Ella Wheeler Wilcox

This handbook contains information about what to do about insomnia, why these strategies work, and how to use them. I will also touch on some of the things you may, or may not, have tried that don't work and explain why they are unhelpful. In addition, to promote your active engagement with the material in the handbook, and to ensure you get maximum benefit from learning and applying the strategies, there are written activities throughout the handbook for you to complete. At this point, this might sound like homework, but believe me, these activities will help you understand how all of this applies to you as an individual and these insights are going to help you conquer your insomnia. Therefore, it will be worth it when you start to see the results. That being said, results will not be achieved straight away.

As a well known hair product commercial stated: "It won't happen overnight, but it will happen." Insomnia doesn't develop overnight. Months or years of poor sleep patterns likewise do not usually develop overnight. It would also be unrealistic to expect that your chronic insomnia would be resolved overnight. Expecting quick fixes is what gets you into trouble with issues like sedative dependence (more on that later). There is no quick fix for insomnia but there is a slow fix – you must be patient and persevere. Then you WILL beat it.

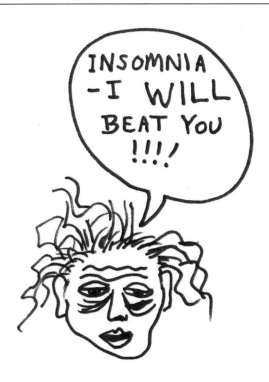

Chapter 1

NORMAL SLEEP

*Now, blessings light on him that first invented sleep! It covers a man
all over, thoughts and all, like a cloak; it is meat for the hungry, drink for
the thirsty, heat for the cold, and cold for the hot. It is the current coin
that purchases all the pleasures of the world cheap, and the balance that
sets the king and the shepherd, the fool and the wise man, even.*
- Miguel de Cervantes, Don Quixote, 1605

INTRODUCTION

In this chapter, I will outline what normal sleep looks like, and how it
varies. You will see that there is enormous variation in the sleep requirements
and sleep habits of individuals. You will also learn that sleep is quite complex,
comprised of several different stages and influenced by many naturally
produced bio-chemicals. I will show you how the circadian cycle and human
body clock work to regulate your sleep-wake patterns. I will also explain the
term, 'sleep debt' and show you how your body deals with it.

SLEEP IS NOT ONE SINGLE STATE

Although it may sometimes seem like one solid single state, normal sleep
is actually made up of different types of sleep that are quite distinct from one
another. Sleep is divided into non–rapid eye movement (NREM) and rapid eye
movement (REM) sleep. There are progressively deeper stages of NREM

sleep, characterized by lower frequency, higher amplitude brain waves as we fall deeper into sleep.

The lightest stage of sleep, Stage 1 is composed mostly of alpha waves. This light phase of sleep often occurs in the transition between wake and sleep and also during short arousal periods during sleep. It accounts for about two to five percent of overall sleep time. The next deepest stage, Stage 2, consists mainly of theta waves, and is the part of sleep where we spend the most time (around 45 to 55% of total sleep).

The deepest stages of NREM sleep, Stages 3 and 4, are made up mainly of delta waves, taking up about five to fifteen percent of overall sleep time. When a person is in this deepest stage of sleep, they are quite difficult to rouse and can be a little disoriented and drowsy after being woken.

REM sleep is completely different from NREM sleep and during this type of sleep, the brain is actually very active. The beta brain waves that occur during REM sleep appear very similar to the brain activity that occurs during waking. Over the course of a typical 8-hour sleep, REM sleep occurs four to five times, with the first REM period lasting for less than 10 minutes, lengthening with each successive REM period, until the duration of the last REM period is usually more than an hour. Over the course of a night, REM sleep takes up about 20 to 25% of total sleep time.

During the night, most people progress through several sleep cycles, with each cycle consisting of light sleep progressing to deeper NREM sleep, followed by a period of REM sleep. The sleep cycles tend to be shorter in the initial parts of the night, lasting around 70 to 100 minutes. Later in the night, the cycles may last for around one and a half to two hours.

As the night goes on, the composition of these cycles usually progressively changes, with more deep, slow-wave, NREM sleep occurring early in the night and more REM sleep occurring towards morning. The make-up of the sleep structure throughout the night is called "sleep architecture" (see Figure 1), probably because it looks a little like a row of skyscrapers when it is mapped out on a hypnogram (a graph which maps sleep stages across time), as they have been measured on an electroencephalograph or EEG.

WHAT KIND OF SLEEP IS MOST IMPORTANT?

Research seems to point to all sleep stages being important, but when push comes to shove, the human brain seems to put slow-wave sleep, our deepest sleep, at the highest priority. For example, if research participants are deliberately deprived of sleep for a few nights in a row, they will 'catch up' on extra slow-wave sleep, before catching up on REM sleep or lighter non-REM sleep. Some people naturally require less sleep than others.

SHORT SLEEPERS VS LONG SLEEPERS

An interesting study by Aeschbach in 1996 showed that habitual short sleepers (those who require an average of less than six hours of sleep each night) need to catch up on less slow-wave sleep after having their sleep restricted than long sleepers (those who normally require nine or more hours of sleep per night). Furthermore, although long sleepers slept for 50% longer than short sleepers, both groups had similar amounts of slow-wave sleep. In other words, it seems that short sleepers have a more 'concentrated' sleep and therefore tolerate sleep loss better.

HOW THE CIRCADIAN RHYTHM INFLUENCES SLEEP

The circadian rhythm is one of several intrinsic body rhythms that are governed by different parts of the hypothalamus in the brain. A pair of tiny, pin-head-sized structures, called the suprachiasmatic nuclei (SCN), in the hypothalamus, are responsible for setting our "body clocks" to a daily cycle which is a little longer than 24 hours. Why the cycle isn't exactly 24 hours is a mystery.

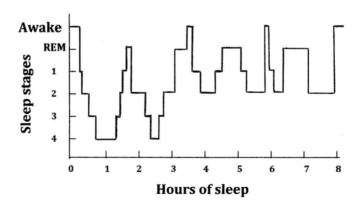

Figure 1. The sleep architecture of a typical night's sleep.

When this circadian cycle is upset by long-distance travel (jet lag), imposed isolation or shift work, the SCN attempts to re-set itself, guided mainly by outside cues such as light, physical activity, noise and temperature. These cues are called *zeitgebers*, a German word meaning time-givers. Light cues are particularly important and messages about the amount of light around us is transmitted by the optic nerves from the eyes to the SCN.

The SCN then transmits information about the time of day to other parts of the brain and subsequently, hormones such as melatonin, growth hormone, prolactin and testosterone, are released in particular quantities appropriate to the perceived time of day. For example: Melatonin (which is secreted by the pineal gland and induces sleepiness) is released as darkness falls; growth hormone (which helps growth and tissue repair) is released at its highest levels during deep sleep; and cortisol is secreted at its highest levels in the morning just prior to awakening in readiness for the physical demands of the day.

Body temperature cycles also mirror the circadian cycle and are regulated by the hypothalamus. Body temperature decreases during the night and sleep deprived animals have difficulty regulating their body temperature.

WHAT IS A NORMAL BED TIME?

It is believed that individuals are genetically programmed to prefer either a late or early bedtime and waking time. Although most adolescents tend to prefer to rise and go to bed late, they tend to outgrow this as adults and settle into a pattern that fits in with their adult schedules. Having small children in the house can also change our natural sleeping habits. However, on weekends or when you are on vacation, you may notice that you settle into your natural rhythm.

HOW MUCH SLEEP DO WE NEED?

There is no magic number! While it is commonly believed that we should all have 8 hours of sleep per night, research indicates optimal adult sleeping habits can vary from 5 to 10 hours per night, depending upon the individual. Most people find that they need slightly less sleep as they get older, and this is a normal part of aging.

WHAT KIND OF BIRD ARE YOU?

The University of Surrey's School of Biomedical and Molecular Sciences has a center for the study of chronobiology, or biological cycles. Researchers there have investigated individual differences in people's circadian clocks and they found distinct differences in the circadian rhythms of study participants, with "larks" going to bed early, getting up earlier and being more alert in the mornings, and "owls" staying up late, waking up later and feeling more alert at night. The study showed that genetic predisposition played an important role in determining whether a person is an early bird or a night owl.

When we have had the optimal amount of sleep, we can go through the next day without feeling sleepy. If tiredness is affecting your ability to do everyday activities, it is possible that you are not getting enough good quality sleep. There is wide variation in the amount of sleep that individuals require, and therefore there is usually no need for concern if you seem to require less or more sleep than other people you know.

AN EXTREME CASE OF HEALTHY INSOMNIA

Research conducted in the early 1970s by Meddis, Pearson and Langford (1973) examined the case of a 70-year old retired nurse who claimed to need only one hour of sleep each night. She did not nap during the day and reported that she filled the time she saved by not sleeping with writing and painting. Meddis had her complete a sleep log for 2 weeks and this showed she was sleeping for an average of 49 minutes per night. It is not uncommon for individuals to come forward with such claims, so Meddis observed the woman sleeping over five nights in the sleep laboratory while she was connected to an electroencephalograph (EEG) machine to record her brain wave activity. She was found to sleep between zero and 3 ½ hours per night, averaging 67 minutes per night over the five-night study period. The study verified her claim and also showed that almost half of her sleep was taken up with slow-wave (deep) sleep, unusual for a woman of this age, confirming the brain's tendency to prioritize slow-wave sleep over other types of sleep. The woman was apparently healthy.

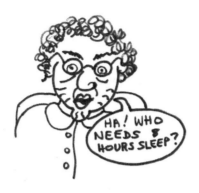

HOW MUCH SLEEP DO MOST PEOPLE HAVE?

Recommended sleep amounts vary depending on age, as does the amount of time people actually regularly sleep. For adults the average daily sleep requirement is around 7.5 hours per night, but according to a National Sleep Foundation Poll in 2003, the average regular amount achieved by adults is 6.99 hours per night. The difference between these two numbers tells us that on average adults are not getting as much sleep as they probably need.

Sleep tends to become lighter with age, and consequently older adults are likely to wake up more often during the night than younger adults. It's helpful to remember that some people naturally need less than 7.5 hours sleep, while others naturally need more than 7.5 hours, so you should not be concerned if your sleep time varies somewhat from this.

POWERFUL SHORT (AND LONG) SLEEPERS

Some powerful public figures famously slept for quite short periods on a regular basis. Winston Churchill slept for only six hours per night (but he also suffered from depression and napped for up to two hours every afternoon!) Margaret Thatcher cultivated a habit of only sleeping for four hours per night (she generally had one night per week when she repaid her sleep debt). Bill Clinton got by on five to six hours sleep per night and Thomas Edison only needed four to six hours (although he was also known to nap). On the other hand, Albert Einstein preferred to get around ten hours of sleep each night.

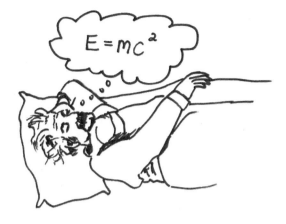

IS THERE SUCH A THING AS TOO MUCH SLEEP?

While too little sleep can have effects on one's physical and mental wellbeing, too much sleep can also sometimes be associated with poor health. Furthermore, the excessive sleep may be of poor quality. In these cases, there is usually another factor at work. For example, people with obstructive sleep apnea seem to sleep at night as well as nap frequently during the day. However, their sleep is in fact of very poor quality, due to frequent interruptions caused by obstructed breathing.

DOES YOUR BODY NEED TO MAKE UP THE SLEEP YOU HAVE LOST?

When a person has experienced several poor nights of sleep in succession, they may start to accumulate a *sleep debt*. Think of your sleep like money and your body like a bank. If you take too much out of your sleep "account" by not getting enough sleep, you have a debt – in other words, you "owe" sleep to your body. Your body is much kinder than most banks though – it doesn't demand that you pay back all you owe, only some of it. For example, if you lose seven hours sleep, it may only take an extra hour or two over one night to make up for this loss.

It is extremely rare for people to take more than three days of good sleep to make up for lost sleep. One good thing to remember is that a little bit of sleep debt is not necessarily a bad thing, because the body is actually good at "calling in" the debt, and we tend to sleep better on nights when we owe some sleep to our bodies.

For the most part, the human brain seems to be very efficient at ensuring we get the rest we need. However, sometimes when sleep loss has been chronic, and the debt is not repaid, the body may try to make up for the debt in other ways, such as physical illness, depressed mood or severe fatigue.

After months or years of disturbed or disrupted sleep, it can take several weeks to re-establish good sleeping patterns. This process requires patience, commitment and perseverance, but it is well worth the effort. As you start using the techniques found in this book, remember that it will take time for your sleep to be established in a better routine.

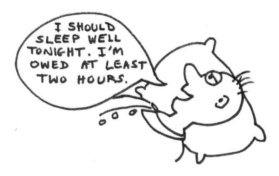

HOW OFTEN DO MOST PEOPLE WAKE UP AT NIGHT?

It's often hard to tell how many times you wake up during the night, especially if it's only for a minute or two. Studies show that we all wake briefly several times per night, but we tend to forget most of these awakenings by morning. In general, the older a person gets the more they will wake up at night.

People aged in their 50s and 60s are typically aware of waking up between one and two times per night. On average, people 70 and over report they wake up between two and three times per night. However, there are lots of people who wake up less or more than this.

Last night I dreamed I had insomnia. I woke up exhausted, yet too well rested to go back to sleep.

- Bob Ingman

Some people are more prone to being aware of even brief awakenings and some are more likely to remember the awakenings in the morning. It is likely that Bob Ingman was one of these people, although he did at least recognize that he was well rested so really knew he had in fact slept normally. Such people may sometimes, however, get the impression that they are sleeping poorly when in fact they may be waking no more frequently than others.

It's important to remember if you do wake up at night, that you should avoid becoming anxious about it. Worrying about being awake during the night can just make it harder to get back to sleep. If you look at the normal pattern of sleep architecture in Figure 1, you can see that it is quite normal to be awake a few times during the night.

CONCLUSION

In this chapter, I have explained the basics of what normal sleep looks like and shown that it is a reasonably complex phenomenon, although most aspects of sleep occur without our awareness. I have also shown that what might be normal for one person is not necessarily normal for others and there is quite a lot of variation in individuals' sleep patterns and behaviors. Hopefully, I have deconstructed some of the myths that you may have heard about sleep and insomnia, so that you can proceed with the strategies outlined in this book with a little less anxiety.

REFERENCE

Meddis, R., Pearson, A. J. & Langford, G. (1973). An extreme case of healthy insomnia. *Electroencephalography and Clinical Neurophysiology*, *35* (2), 213-214.

Chapter 2

YOUR SLEEP ASSESSMENT

INTRODUCTION

This chapter contains some sleep assessments for you to complete and this will help to give you a base-line measure of where your sleep, sleep patterns and associated thinking are at right now. Make a blank copy of these questionnaires before you start using the approaches outlined in this handbook, or complete the scales below in pencil, so that if you need to complete them again in the future, you can. You will need to score these questionnaires yourself and instructions will be given to help you do that. You should answer the questions in relation to how you have felt, thought, slept and behaved over the past month only and your answers should relate to the majority of the time in that month.

Please answer as carefully and accurately as you can. It is common for people who have suffered from insomnia for a long time to over-rate their symptoms on scales such as these. This is because they may feel that others don't properly appreciate the distress the insomnia causes them and that showing other people a high score on an actual questionnaire will "prove" how bad they feel. Try to avoid the urge to over-rate your symptoms in this way. On the other hand, don't under-rate your symptoms either. Be as accurate as possible. No matter how high your scores are, the strategies described in this handbook should still help you resolve your insomnia, provided that you are willing, consistent and patient about putting them into practice.

Here's another tip: Please don't complete these questionnaires in the evening right before going to bed, or you may find that doing so creates counter-productive worry and stress about your insomnia.

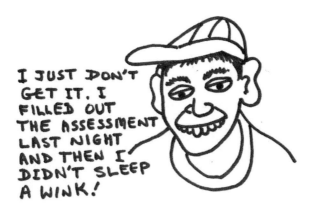

MEASURE 1: SLEEP PATTERNS AND HABITS

Complete the following questionnaire to give yourself a baseline regarding your normal sleep patterns.

1. How many hours of sleep did you get on average each night when you were a young adult?
    _____hours
2. How many hours of sleep do you estimate that you currently get on average each night, in total?
    _____hours
3. How many hours of sleep do you feel you need per night?
    _____hours
4. Is your sleep disturbed at night?   Yes   No
    If you answered yes, describe how your sleep is disturbed, how frequently and for how long each night?

    _____

    _____

5. What is your normal bedtime? If it varies, what is the range of usual bedtimes?

    _____

6. What is your normal waking time? If it varies, what is the range of usual waking times?

_____

7. How many minutes, on average, does it take you to fall asleep each night?
_____ mins

8. How many times, on average, do you wake per night and then have difficulty falling back to sleep?

_____

9. Please circle any of the following issues that interrupt your sleep on most nights.

Nightmares   Indigestion/reflux   Restless legs   Snoring
Pain   Breathing difficulties   Temperature   Noise
Pets   Partner's movements/snoring Need to use the bathroom
Other reason/s: _____

10. How many nights, on average, per week, do you take a substance (e.g., alcohol, prescription sedative, herbal sedative) to help you sleep?
_____ nights/week

11. How many days, on average, per week, do you awake feeling unrefreshed by your night's sleep?
_____ days/week

12. How would you rate your sleep quality, in general (please circle one)?

Dreadful   Extremely poor   Poor   Average
Good   Extremely good   Excellent

13. Please circle below which of the following is a problem for you on most nights (circle all that apply).
Having problems falling off to sleep
Having problems staying asleep
Waking up too early and then being unable to go back to sleep

MEASURE 2: TIREDNESS

The following items relate to tiredness and fatigue during the day. Please rate yourself according to the following scale, in relation to the past month.

0 = Never
1 = Occasionally
2 = Regularly
3 = Frequently
4 = Every day

1. I feel fatigued or tired in general.	0	1	2	3	4
2. I feel completely exhausted.	0	1	2	3	4
3. I feel too tired to eat.	0	1	2	3	4
4. I feel too tired to work effectively.	0	1	2	3	4
5. I feel too tired to carry out normal activities.	0	1	2	3	4
6. I feel too tired to drive.	0	1	2	3	4
7. I fall asleep at the wheel of a car.	0	1	2	3	4
8. I fall asleep when a passenger in a car.	0	1	2	3	4
9. I fall asleep on public transport.	0	1	2	3	4
10. I fall asleep while reading at work.	0	1	2	3	4
11. I fall asleep while reading (seated) at home.	0	1	2	3	4
12. I fall asleep watching television.	0	1	2	3	4
13. I fall asleep during conversations.	0	1	2	3	4
14. I am so fatigued that I do not feel safe.	0	1	2	3	4
15. My thinking ability is affected by fatigue.	0	1	2	3	4
16. My concentration is affected by fatigue.	0	1	2	3	4
17. My memory is affected by fatigue.	0	1	2	3	4
18. I fall asleep at the movies.	0	1	2	3	4
19. I fall asleep at the hairdressing salon.	0	1	2	3	4
20. I fall asleep while eating.	0	1	2	3	4
21. I fall asleep while socializing.	0	1	2	3	4
21. My ability to enjoy is affected by fatigue.	0	1	2	3	4
22. My happiness is affected by fatigue.	0	1	2	3	4
23. My energy/liveliness is affected by fatigue.	0	1	2	3	4
24. My motivation is affected by fatigue.	0	1	2	3	4
25. My mood is affected by fatigue.	0	1	2	3	4
26. My ability to cope is affected by fatigue.	0	1	2	3	4
27. My enthusiasm is affected by fatigue.	0	1	2	3	4

28. Getting things done is affected by my fatigue.   0   1   2   3   4
29. My social life is affected by fatigue.   0   1   2   3   4

Sub-total: Add up each column   _   _   _   _   _
Add total score   _____

MEASURE 3: SLEEP-RELATED THINKING AND ACTIONS

The following items relate to sleep-related thinking and actions that you may/may not engage in. Please rate yourself according to the following scale, in relation to the past month.

0 = Never
1 = Occasionally
2 = Regularly
3 = Frequently
4 = Every day

1. I take substances (e.g., alcohol, sedatives)
    to help me sleep   0   1   2   3   4
2. I nap during the day to make up for lost sleep.   0   1   2   3   4
3. I try very hard to sleep well at night.   0   1   2   3   4
4. I rearrange my day to cope with sleep loss.   0   1   2   3   4
5. I check the clock during the night.   0   1   2   3   4
6. I calculate how much sleep I am getting.   0   1   2   3   4
7. I try to keep active so I will sleep better.   0   1   2   3   4
8. I speak to friends and family about my sleep.   0   1   2   3   4
9. I am very conscious of my comfort in bed.   0   1   2   3   4
10. I monitor how much sleep I am missing.   0   1   2   3   4
11. I go to bed later in order to sleep better.   0   1   2   3   4
12. I worry about insomnia and sleep loss.   0   1   2   3   4
13. I feel anxious because of sleep loss.   0   1   2   3   4
14. I feel moody because of sleep loss.   0   1   2   3   4
15. I am easily irritated because of sleep loss.   0   1   2   3   4
16. I snap at others because of tiredness.   0   1   2   3   4
17. I feel hopeless about my sleep.   0   1   2   3   4
18. I think I will never be able to sleep without
    something to sedate me.   0   1   2   3   4

19. I feel frustrated that I cannot control my sleep.	0	1	2	3	4
20. I feel nervous about going to bed.	0	1	2	3	4
21. I lack confidence in my ability to sleep well.	0	1	2	3	4
22. I doubt I will ever sleep well.	0	1	2	3	4
23. I know I will be unable to function properly if I don't get a good nights sleep.	0	1	2	3	4
24. I feel the need to catch up on lost sleep.	0	1	2	3	4
25. I worry about the health impact of sleep loss.	0	1	2	3	4
26. I worry about not getting 8 hours of sleep.	0	1	2	3	4
27. I always need at least 8 hours sleep per night.	0	1	2	3	4
28. I worry about having nightmares.	0	1	2	3	4
29. I tend to worry about many things.	0	1	2	3	4
30. I feel overwhelmed with worry and stress.	0	1	2	3	4
31. I worry more than I used to.	0	1	2	3	4
32. I worry about the impact of sleep loss on my daily functioning.	0	1	2	3	4
33. I worry about my inability to control my sleep.	0	1	2	3	4
34. Rather than be tired the next day, I tend to take a sedative.	0	1	2	3	4
35. When I am anxious or stressed, I feel it is due to poor sleep.	0	1	2	3	4
36. When I feel depressed, I feel it is due to poor sleep.	0	1	2	3	4
37. When I lack energy or motivation, I feel it is due to poor sleep.	0	1	2	3	4
38. I tend to stay home after a night of poor sleep.	0	1	2	3	4
39. I avoid work after a night of poor sleep.	0	1	2	3	4
Add up each column	–	–	–	–	–
Add total score	____				

Now add your total scores from each of the measures and keep a record of this score for comparison purposes after you have applied the strategies outlined in this book. This, along with the sleep diary information (see the following pages) gives you some good baseline information about your overall sleep patterns. The next chapter explains why we sleep and how the different stages of sleep are thought to serve different functions.

INSTRUCTIONS FOR KEEPING THE WEEKLY SLEEP DIARY

1. Do not complete this during the night, but rather do it in the morning.

2. Keep the sleep diary for at least 2 weeks prior to starting to use the strategies outlined in this book. Then keep the sleep diary for at least 4 weeks while you are putting the strategies into practice. However, you will have to estimate any times that you were awake at night because one of the strategies is to not look at the clock overnight. Do not keep a sleep diary for any longer because it can become counter-productive to focus too much on measuring your sleep.

3. Write in the day, day of the week, and whether the day was a work day, day off or vacation day.

4. Put a line (I) to indicate when you went to bed.

5. Shade in all boxes to show that you were asleep, including times that you napped during the day.

6. Leave boxes un-shaded to indicate that you were awake at those times (night or day).

7. Place a dot (.) to indicate when you take any sedative medication.

8. An alternative to keeping the sleep diary is to use a sleep measuring app (see Appendix 1 for a list and description of some of these, such as Sleep Cycle and SleepBot) on your smart phone to monitor your nightly sleep patterns. The advantage of this approach is that you are not so involved yourself in measuring and paying attention to your sleep loss and focusing on the distress caused by it. These apps also provide you with objective sleep graphs and sound recordings.

Weekly Sleep Diary

Date	Day of Week	Type of Day	12md	1pm	2pm	3pm	4pm	5pm	6pm	7pm	8pm	9pm	10pm	11pm	12mn	1am	2am	3am	4am	5am	6am	7am	8am	9am	10am	11am
Example	Thurs	Work							■			I		■	■	■		■	■	■	■					

Weekly Sleep Diary

Date	Day of Week	Type of Day	12md	1pm	2pm	3pm	4pm	5pm	6pm	7pm	8pm	9pm	10pm	11pm	12mn	1am	2am	3am	4am	5am	6am	7am	8am	9am	10am	11am
Example	Thurs	Work							■			I		■	■	■		■	■	■	■					

Weekly Sleep Diary

Date	Day of Week	Type of Day	12pm	1pm	2pm	3pm	4pm	5pm	6pm	7pm	8pm	9pm	10pm	11pm	12mn	1am	2am	3am	4am	5am	6am	7am	8am	9am	10am	11am
Example	Thurs	Work							▓			I		▓	▓	▓		▓	▓	▓	▓					

Weekly Sleep Diary

Date	Day of Week	Type of Day	12pm	1pm	2pm	3pm	4pm	5pm	6pm	7pm	8pm	9pm	10pm	11pm	12mn	1am	2am	3am	4am	5am	6am	7am	8am	9am	10am	11am
Example	Thurs	Work							▓			I		▓	▓	▓		▓	▓	▓	▓					

Weekly Sleep Diary

Date	Day of Week	Type of Day	12md	1pm	2pm	3pm	4pm	5pm	6pm	7pm	8pm	9pm	10pm	11pm	12mn	1am	2am	3am	4am	5am	6am	7am	8am	9am	10am	11am
Example	Thurs	Work							▓			I		▓	▓	▓		▓	▓	▓	▓					

Weekly Sleep Diary

Date	Day of Week	Type of Day	12md	1pm	2pm	3pm	4pm	5pm	6pm	7pm	8pm	9pm	10pm	11pm	12mn	1am	2am	3am	4am	5am	6am	7am	8am	9am	10am	11am
Example	Thurs	Work							▓			I		▓	▓	▓		▓	▓	▓	▓					

Weekly Sleep Diary

Date	Day of Week	Type of Day	12md	1pm	2pm	3pm	4pm	5pm	6pm	7pm	8pm	9pm	10pm	11pm	12mn	1am	2am	3am	4am	5am	6am	7am	8am	9am	10am	11am
Example	Thurs	Work							▓			I		▓	▓	▓		▓	▓	▓	▓					

Chapter 3

WHY DO WE SLEEP?

Sleep is the best meditation

- Dalai Lama

INTRODUCTION

If you have ever missed a night's sleep you may have experienced a feeling of being so tired that it seemed you weren't functioning properly. For most of us, feelings like this intuitively tell us that sleep is important. We spend roughly a third of our lives asleep, which amounts to around 26 years in total for an average Westerner! That's a lot of time to be spending doing something that has no good purpose.

In this chapter, I will outline the main scientific theories that have been put forward to explain why we sleep and what might be occurring in each of the different stages of sleep. You will see that sleep remains a mystery, even to those who have been studying the phenomenon for decades. You will also learn about the main theories that have been developed to explain why we dream.

DO WE REALLY NEED TO SLEEP AT ALL?

Imagine what you could do with all that time if you didn't need to sleep. Yet most of us actually wouldn't want to dispense with sleep – it is something we enjoy and even look forward to. It is a pleasurable experience, so long as it is working normally for us.

Even though we don't fully understand what its purpose is, we want to have a full night's sleep and that is because we all have an innate drive to sleep, similar to our drive to eat, drink and have sex. However, it is probably more powerful than almost all of these other drives. Only our drive to consume fluid is comparable.

There are several theories about why we sleep but surprisingly, even with all the science and studies of sleep over the past century, nothing has been proven conclusively and the full purpose of sleep remains in essence, a mystery. No single unifying theory has been shown to explain the full purpose of sleep. Sleep probably serves many functions and therefore, many of the theories relating to the purpose of sleep are possibly all correct at the same time.

> *People say, 'I'm going to sleep now,' as if it were nothing. But it's really a bizarre activity. 'For the next several hours, while the sun is gone, I'm going to become unconscious, temporarily losing command over everything I know and understand. When the sun returns, I will resume my life.' If you didn't know what sleep was, and you had only seen it in a science fiction movie, you would think it was weird and tell all your friends about the movie you'd seen. They had these people, you know? And they would walk around all day and be OK? And then, once a day, usually after dark, they would lie down on these special platforms and become unconscious. They would stop functioning almost completely, except deep in their minds they would have adventures and experiences that were completely impossible in real life.*
> – George Carlin, Brain Droppings

George Carlin really has a good point here. Sleep is really a very strange activity when you think about it. It doesn't seem to have any obvious purpose and in some ways, it seems like a sort of evolutionary hangover from our prehistoric humanoid ancestors. Even for them, it would have been pretty unhelpful and would have made them vulnerable to predators at night.

Many theories about the function of sleep are based on the evolution of sleep in humans and other animals. We know that all mammals, amphibians, reptiles, birds and even fish sleep. For some animals, sleeping poses a significant risk because during this time, they are vulnerable to attack from predators. Even dolphins, that would drown if they slept in the same way as land mammals, have evolved an incredible adaptation whereby one hemisphere of their brain remains awake while the other sleeps, so that they can continue to surface and breathe.

Adaptations such as this do not occur in nature through evolution unless there are important reasons for them to do so. From this we can deduce that sleep serves some important purpose or purposes that somehow aid in the survival of these species.

> *It's in the morning, for most of us. It's that time, those few seconds when we're coming out of sleep but we're not really awake yet. For those few seconds we're something more primitive than what we are about to become. We have just slept the sleep of our most distant ancestors, and something of them and their world still clings to us.*
>
> – Jerry Spinelli, Stargirl

Theories that fit well with the idea that sleep is somehow adaptive and helpful to our survival as a species include the conservation theory, the inactivity theory, and the restoration theory.

CONSERVATION THEORY

This theory proposes that sleep serves to help the body to conserve energy for a period each day by keeping it relatively still. Also during sleep, we are not engaged in consuming food or (particularly in our ancestors' times) foraging or hunting for food, at night when we would be least likely to be successful in such efforts.

Even in modern times, we do consume less energy when we are asleep, partly because we move less and partly because our body temperature is reduced. In addition, certain hunger-regulating hormones are secreted at different levels during sleep than during wakefulness. Through the suppression of hunger that occurs during sleep, we conserve our food resources.

Evolution presumably dictated that amongst our early predecessors, those who slept for an optimal length of time during dark hours and hunted and foraged for a maximal length of time during daylight hours were selected by nature over many millennia for survival and reproduction. Interestingly, some studies more recently have suggested that modern humans sleep for roughly an hour less per night than they did in Victorian times, which is only about 120 years ago.

The invention of artificial light has fundamentally changed an important factor impacting on our sleep patterns and this has occurred over a relatively short period of time in evolutionary terms. Whether this shortening of our sleep patterns turns out to be helpful to our survival or not will be determined over time and it is much too soon to tell.

INACTIVITY THEORY

The inactivity theory suggests that sleep keeps us in one place when it is dark and potentially an unsafe time for us to be moving about very much and risking falling or being attacked by nocturnal predators. In other words, this theory suggests that sleep may have evolved out of a risk minimization strategy of staying still and quiet and out of harm's way during a high-risk time of each 24-hour period. By having fewer accidents and attacks from predators, certain ancestors of ours may have been naturally selected to be stronger, healthier and more likely to survive and reproduce and pass on the same strategies to their young.

Eventually, most probably in a very primitive prehistoric, pre-mammalian ancestor, this inactive phase may have evolved into what we actually now experience as sleep. The main weakness in this theory is that we are less vigilant when we are asleep and being so inactive whilst asleep that we are relatively unconscious poses certain risks as well.

RESTORATION THEORY

There is no doubt that we generally feel physically restored after a good night's sleep. Sleep allows us to rest our bodies completely so that they can function optimally the following day. But why does this restful state give us this sense of restoration? Sleep creates the optimal conditions for cellular healing and growth. Indeed, growth hormone is secreted at peak levels during sleep. We do know from sleep deprivation experiments that when animals are prevented from sleeping, their immunity suffers and they die within only a few weeks.

Although such experiments have been carried out with rats and mice in the past, it is no longer considered ethical and would never be allowed in humans. However, there have been cases where individuals attempted to stay awake in order to break records. Even with whole teams of people devoted to the task of keeping one person awake, it has never been possible to keep a person awake for more than 11 days – after this time, the person begins to enter sleep states whilst appearing to be awake and micro-sleeps become impossible to prevent.

LEARNING AND BRAIN DEVELOPMENT THEORIES

Beyond these 'physical conservation and restoration' theories, there are also theories that suggest at least part of the reason we sleep is to sustain a state which is optimal for certain kinds of brain activity to occur. Young animals, such as human infants, sleep a great deal more than adults, which suggests that sleep is highly correlated with brain development. Other studies suggest that adult animals including human adults sleep more during periods of increased learning. Still other studies have suggested that certain kinds of learning are improved by increasing sleep.

Any or all of these theories relating to the reasons why we sleep, and why we need to sleep, could constitute the factual basis for why many animals, including humans, have evolved to require sleep. There is no doubt that we need to sleep and it is actually very difficult to deprive an individual of sleep for any more than a couple of days. Perhaps the best case example of the link between learning and sleep is what research has been able to reveal about some of the functions of Rapid Eye Movement (REM) sleep.

REM SLEEP AND LEARNING

There are several pieces of evidence that all point to REM sleep having its own function and evolutionary adaptive advantage. These include: the great difficulties encountered when experimental attempts are made to selectively deprive humans and other animals of REM sleep; the phenomenon of REM rebound following periods of REM deprivation; and the evolutionary evidence, suggesting that REM sleep has persisted in terrestrial mammalian species for at least 40 million years. Evolutionary design tends to dispense with animal behaviors that don't have some sort of adaptive value, so we can assume that REM sleep gives us a definite edge in terms of survival.

The available evidence suggests that, during REM sleep, the human brain uses more energy, in the form of oxygen and glucose, than during the waking state. When you look at human brain activity on an electroencephalogram (EEG), the electrical activity of REM sleep appears quite similar to how it would appear if the person was awake. The brain waves are mainly high frequency and low amplitude waves.

Animal studies have demonstrated an important role of REM sleep in learning and memory formation and some evidence has been found to suggest that complex, procedural learning is somehow consolidated during REM sleep. Some studies have suggested that a combination of slow-wave sleep followed by REM sleep may be required for the processing of procedural memories.

Neuroimaging studies have shown that the limbic and paralimbic forebrain structures of the brain are particularly active during REM sleep and the activation of these particular areas suggests that motivational and emotional learning may also be processed during this stage of sleep. This may account for why REM sleep dreams can be so intense and emotional.

The accumulation of studies seems to suggest that *procedural memory* (the ability to perform particular tasks) is dependent on REM sleep but *declarative memory* (knowledge of facts) is facilitated more by Slow Wave Sleep. Like the waking state, REM sleep is actually a very complex state of consciousness, which probably serves many functions and facilitates many processes.

AN INTERESTING FACT ABOUT REM SLEEP

During REM sleep, the brain's cortex is still producing motor commands, but due to an inhibitory mechanism that blocks activity in the spinal cord, we are completely paralyzed. We can move our eyes and our involuntary muscles keep us breathing, but we are effectively as if we had been shot with a tranquillizer dart.

The mechanism that causes this paralysis lies in the base of our brains, and Italian experiments on cats in the 1960s showed that when this mechanism was physically destroyed, the animals moved around during REM sleep as if they were "acting out" their dreams. They prowled around the laboratory, arched their backs, and pursued imaginary prey, all with barely a sound and all whilst sound asleep.

It seems that the purpose of the paralysis mechanism is to prevent us from acting out our dreams and coming to some sort of harm in the process. Indeed, there is a rare human disorder, REM Behavior Disorder, where sufferers do act out their dreams, frequently resulting in serious injuries to both the sufferers and their sleeping partners!

It certainly seems that mammals have evolved to ensure that we cannot execute the commands to our motor systems that our dreaming brains are sending. Although there are differences between individuals in how complete the resulting muscle atonia is, most skeletal muscle tone is considerably reduced, effectively paralyzing the individual.

WHEN DO WE DREAM?

Although dreaming is more characteristic of REM sleep than other sleep stages, it turns out that is not exclusively confined to any particular stage of sleep. It is now well-documented that dreams can also take place as we are nodding off, in non-REM sleep, and even in relaxed waking states. Nevertheless, it is well established that dream recall is highest following awakening from REM sleep (around 81.8%), compared to non-REM sleep (around 42.5%).

Of course, it is possible that we dream continuously throughout all stages of sleep, but that amnesia of our dreams is more likely in the deeper stages. Indeed there is abundant evidence that dreams occur even during general anesthesia and deep coma, although memories of them tend to decay very rapidly.

While REM sleep may be the state of consciousness that is most conducive to dreaming, dreaming and REM sleep are still not quite the same thing. Dreaming can occur in the absence of REM sleep, and that REM sleep can occur without dreaming.

WHY DO WE DREAM?

Every night, almost every human on the planet spends between one and two hours in REM sleep. And although we often don't remember the details, we spend most of this time dreaming. We know that dreams are different from waking consciousness and that unlike waking fantasies or daydreams, we feel that dreams happen to us, rather than as a direct result of our own will.

Dreams often contain bizarre and impossible events – we fly, we fight dinosaurs, and we watch without horror as familiar people morph into animals

– we don't seem to be able to predict or anticipate the content of these nightly hallucinations. It is perhaps this suspension of logic and the knowledge that our minds are unconsciously producing these imaginings that makes them so fascinating to us.

> *Even a soul submerged in sleep is hard at work and helps make something of the world.*
>
>   – Heraclitus, Fragments

Dreams, along with their origins and meanings, have preoccupied humankind since the earliest times. Even today, many tribal societies regard dreams as central to their understanding of the world and their place in it. Interest in dreams and their meaning is alive and well in Western societies too, where many individuals enjoy sharing their dreams and pondering their significance with others.

Many books have been written about interpreting dreams, and sometimes it is difficult to distinguish fiction and speculation from scientific fact. In actuality, dreams have been extensively studied for over 50 years and there is even an international scientific body devoted to the study of dreaming, the Association for the Study of Dreams.

Dreams are awkward to study, mainly because of their personal and subjective nature, and the fact that they occur while we are asleep and are so easily forgotten. Although Freud had earlier popularized an interest in dream function and interpretation, it was the advent of the sleep laboratory and the discovery in 1953 of REM sleep that first brought the study of dreaming into the scientific realm.

It would be easy, on the basis of the scientific evidence available, to discount the possibility that dreams serve any real purpose were it not for the intriguing fact that we are completely paralyzed during REM sleep.

If dreaming has no specific purpose, it seems strange that mammals would have evolved such a sophisticated mechanism for dealing with the problem of us potentially acting out our dreams, since nature does not usually go to such lengths to preserve a behavior that has no purpose. And if it is only REM sleep that has important functions, why couldn't it get on with them without the need for dreaming? What's more, dreams can sometimes even interrupt REM sleep, such as when nightmares wake us.

SLEEP-TIME DAY-DREAMING?

What is known about the workings of REM sleep in fact reveals little about dreaming, or about whether dreaming serves any purpose at all. Although dreaming most often occurs in synchrony with the physical state of REM sleep, dreams may not necessarily tell us much about what mental processes are taking place during REM sleep. As John Antrobus, a professor at the University of British Columbia, who specializes in dream research has pointed out, the daydreams of a commuter do not help describe the thinking processes involved in driving a car.

There is now good evidence that REM sleep is important for our learning of complex information and for using insight in problem-solving, and it probably plays a role in the processing of memories. However, the fact that REM sleep has an important purpose does not necessarily mean that dreaming does too, even while dreams may give some indication of the type of work that REM sleep may be doing.

It is a common experience that a problem difficult at night is resolved in the morning after the committee of sleep has worked on it.
- John Steinbeck

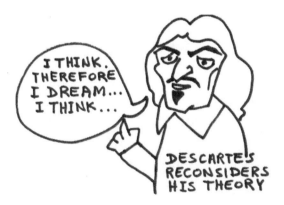

PRACTICING FOR DEALING WITH THREATS?

A popular current theory of why we dream suggests that dreams may help us to adapt to what life throws at us by creating special connections between current stressors and remote memories. Another theory is that we rehearse dealing with threats (for example, fighting off attackers) during dreams to enhance our survival.

Finnish researcher, Anti Revonsuo believes that this is why we tend to dream of spiders, snakes, falling, and being chased by strangers and animals, since these would have been long-standing threats to our ancestors, and might be "pre-programmed" into our psyches. There are doubters of such theories, such as Mark Blagrove, of the University of Wales, who suggest that dreams may have no purpose at all, and may be simply a by-product of a busy brain during REM sleep. What is clear from dream research is that we tend to dream about what concerns us, particularly on an emotional level. An important question, though, is: Does dreaming about what stresses us represent our minds working to resolve these issues or is such dreaming merely symptomatic of our distress? The re-experiencing of trauma in dreams, as in therapy, may or may not be helpful to the dreamer. While some researchers have suggested that dreams might help us to work through emotional problems, there are several difficulties for this hypothesis; including the fact that we remember so few of our dreams and so many that we do remember are completely unrelated to our waking problems. Another problem is that sufferers of post-traumatic stress disorder frequently experience nightmares that tend to make them feel worse rather than better.

CONCLUSION

With all our elaborate sleep laboratories and scientific instruments and theories, we are hardly any closer to understanding dreaming than we were in Freud's day, or even Aristotle's. Although we may sense meaning in our dreams, and while they may fascinate us, we have been unable to define any particular reason for why we experience them. By the same token, sleep and its functions still remain largely a mystery, although there are some clues to its purpose and we definitely know that we can't do without it.

ACTIVITY

1. Now that you have read about the main scientific theories that explain why we sleep, write here what theory/theories make the most sense to you, based on your own personal experiences.

_____

_____

_____

_____

2. Describe the most interesting dream that you have had and what meaning, if any, the dream had for you.

    _____

    _____

    _____

    _____

3. Which theory of dreaming makes the most sense to you, given your own experiences?

    _____

    _____

    _____

    _____

Chapter 4

WHAT IS INSOMNIA?

Then night came down like the feathery soot of a smoky lamp, and smutted first the bed quilt, then the hearth-rug, then the window-seat, and then at last the great, stormy, faraway outside world. But sleep did not come. Oh, no! Nothing new came at all except that particularly wretched, itching type of insomnia which seems to rip away from one's body the whole kind, protecting skin and expose all the raw, ticklish fretwork of nerves to the mercy of a gritty blanket or a wrinkled sheet.
- Eleanor Hallowell Abbott, Molly Make-Believe

INTRODUCTION

In this chapter, I will describe what insomnia actually is as well as examine different types of insomnia. I will show you how common insomnia is worldwide and discuss the factors that can lead to, and contribute to, insomnia. I will introduce the importance of factors that perpetuate insomnia in the longer term, as these are the very factors that I will focus on in the rest of the chapters in this book.

HOW COMMON IS INSOMNIA?

Sleep loss is a very common problem in the wider community and there is evidence that it is second only to pain in the complaints patients bring to their general practitioners. An international survey, conducted by sleep experts from Canada, Japan and Greece, across 10 different countries on International Sleep well Day (March 21) in 2002 found that 24% of the 35,327 people surveyed reported not sleeping well, 31.6% had insomnia according to the self-reported scale they completed, with another 17.5% considered to have 'sub-threshold insomnia' (Soldatos, et al., 2005). Another study, conducted in Britain, interviewed almost 2000 adults aged 16 to 93 years, and found that 58% had experienced sleep problems on one or more nights in the previous week (Groeger, Zijlstra & Dijk, 2004).

Data collected more recently in the United States suggests a similar pattern there, with one 2012 study finding that 30% of employed civilian adults (approximately 40.6 million workers) reported that they slept for 6 hours or less per day (Centers for Disease Control & Prevention, 2012). Another study found that 29.2% of middle-aged Americans reported experiencing insomnia symptoms almost every night or several times per week (Karlson et al., 2013). Yet another recent, population-based telephone survey found that 27.9% of United States adults felt they were frequently getting insufficient sleep (defined as not getting enough rest or sleep for 14 or more days out of the previous 30 days) (Chapman et al., 2012). A Canadian telephone survey of 2000 adults found that 13.4% of the participants met all the clinical criteria for insomnia (Morin, et al., 2011).

> *Not being able to sleep is terrible. You have the misery of having partied all night... without the satisfaction.*
> - Lynn Johnston

Contemporary lifestyle choices, including the volume of work we do, and the times during which we undertake work and leisure activities, play an important part in sleep. These choices are often the basis of many sleep problems.

> *Am I sleeping? Have I slept at all? This is insomnia.*
> - Chuck Palahniuk, Fight Club

We are not always the best judges of our own sleep patterns. We may feel that we haven't slept much at all, when in fact we have slept for several hours in a 24 hour period. Disrupted sleep or waking up a few times in the night may give rise to the misperception that we have slept very poorly. If we feel tired during the day, we may blame this on sleep loss when other factors such as worry and taking on too many commitments may also be contributing. Waking during the night, even several times, does not automatically mean that you haven't had enough sleep. Of course, worrying about sleeping poorly can contribute to stress and overall arousal, which can in turn lead to further sleep loss.

TYPES OF INSOMNIA

It appears that every man's insomnia is as different from his neighbor's as are their daytime hopes and aspirations.

- F Scott Fitzgerald

A few nights of poor sleep does not constitute a sleep disorder. However, if the problem has gone on for over a month, become chronic, and is causing daytime fatigue and distress, it is probably what could be called Insomnia Disorder. There can be many causes of insomnia and some primary causes must be addressed in addition to addressing the insomnia itself. For example, people with Obstructive Sleep Apnea (OSA) or Restless Leg Syndrome (RLS) can develop insomnia as a result of the repeated awakenings caused by the primary disorder. Even when the primary problem is successfully treated, these people can continue to have a problem with insomnia.

Other people may develop insomnia at quite a young age due to the uncertainty and trauma of living in a violent household. They may get into a habit of being vigilant at night in case of potential abuse. Insomnia can also develop in people who experience a traumatic event in adult life.

Still others may develop insomnia without there being any obvious reason for it. Usually in such cases, there has been some stress, worry or lifestyle change that has precipitated the onset of the insomnia.

CAN INSOMNIA KILL YOU?

There is an extraordinarily rare type of insomnia that can, in fact, be fatal. Fortunately, this is very obviously different to the usual variant of insomnia but it is important to discuss it because its existence has led to the idea that it is possible to die from insomnia. This leads to unnecessary worry and concern in individuals with insomnia. This, like all forms of worry, can make insomnia worse.

Fatal Familial Insomnia (FFI) is an incredibly rare disorder that is usually acquired through an inherited genetic mutation. It can also occur through a spontaneous mutation although this is even more rare. Less than a dozen cases have ever been diagnosed. It is a *prion disease* like Creutzfeld-Jacob Disease, which starts with insomnia and leads to dementia and brain damage. Prions are poorly understood infectious proteins. FFI has no known cure and once symptoms begin, patients with FFI deteriorate quickly and only survive for about 18 months. Onset of the disease is in middle-age, usually around the age of 50, but it has been known to occur in younger adults.

The mutated prion protein that causes FFI has only been found in 40 families worldwide. Today, there are only 25 families left in the world that carry the genetic mutation for FFI: eight are in Germany, five in Italy, four in the USA, two in France, two in Britain, two in Australia, one in Austria and one in Japan.

If your family is one of them, chances are that you would know about it and would have been offered genetic testing. If one parent has the faulty gene, their children each have a 50% risk of inheriting it and developing the disease. These days, with genetic testing and genetic counseling, FFI is likely to become even more rare.

Okay, so now we've got that out of the way, be assured that, unless you are one of the unfortunate handful of people in the world with FFI, insomnia cannot kill you!

INSOMNIA CAUSED BY PHYSICAL HEALTH PROBLEMS

You may be aware that your sleep is disturbed, but that doesn't necessarily mean you suffer from a sleep disorder such as insomnia. It is important to speak to your doctor if you are experiencing sleep loss, just in case there is something else that is triggering the disturbance in your sleep. It is possible to experience sleep loss as a symptom of another condition.

Some of the more common conditions that *might* lead to sleep loss include:

- Thyroid conditions;
- Depression;
- Some types of anxiety disorders;
- Asthma or chronic lung disease;
- Use of some prescription drugs;
- Physical pain, like backache or arthritis;
- Type 2 diabetes;

- Obesity;
- Some heart conditions, such as congestive heart failure;
- Sleep apnea; and
- Periodic Limb Movement Disorder (PLMD), often associated with Restless Leg Syndrome (RLS)

If you have one or more of these conditions, it is important that this central problem is properly treated so that you are better able to achieve good sleep. For example, if you are in a great deal of pain from arthritis when you go to bed, this is obviously not conducive to restful sleep. When such conditions are well managed, you are in a position to benefit most from guidelines for promoting quality sleep.

FACTORS THAT AFFECT SLEEP

There are many factors that impact on sleep quantity and quality, some temporarily and some with the potential to have a more long-lasting impact. You do not have the ability to change all of these factors, but there are many you can work on to prevent insomnia from becoming a chronic or permanent problem.

Some of the most common factors that affect your sleep include:

- Your age: It is generally accepted that sleep tends to become lighter and more fragmented with advancing age. However, some research (e.g., Bastien, Vallieres & Morin, 2001) seems to indicate that increased age is not statistically related to insomnia, and that this connection is actually related to health problems associated with older age. About a third of people over the age of 65 report problems with sleeping, but predictive research has shown that there is no relationship between increased age and sleep problems when we take into account how much *regular exercise* people do and how *socially active* they are.
- Your gender: Women are much more likely to report problems with insomnia than men. This could be related to a number of factors, such as hormonal fluctuations and women's greater tendency to ruminate on stressful concerns.

- Your individual constitution and temperament: Some people are simply more likely to develop insomnia. This applies especially to people who have an anxious disposition.
- Your prior sleep patterns: Previous erratic sleep patterns can make you more vulnerable to developing insomnia.
- Prescription drug use: There are many prescription drugs that can cause insomnia; sometimes dosages or the timing of doses can be adjusted by your physician to reduce their impact.
- Non-prescribed substances: Obviously stimulants of any kind are incompatible with good sleep and these include caffeine and nicotine.
- Lifestyle issues: Factors such as stress, worry, shift work or long working hours can all lead to insomnia.
- Psychological disorders: Anxiety and mood disorders commonly cause sleep difficulties and are sometimes a key symptom. Depression can also result from prolonged periods of insomnia.

THE THREE PS

In general, the factors that can cause or worsen insomnia can be grouped into three types – let's call them the three Ps. These are predisposing factors, precipitating factors and perpetuating factors. Often you will find that you have little or no control over the predisposing and precipitating factors, but you can work on the perpetuating factors to stop your insomnia from taking a permanent hold on your sleep.

PREDISPOSING FACTORS

We are each naturally predisposed to many possible physical problems and disorders. This could be as a result of your genetic make-up, developmental factors that occurred during your childhood, youth or early adulthood, or other components of your physical or neurological chemistry. For example, you may come from a family of light sleepers. Many sleep disorders, such as the parasomnias (including sleep walking), seem to have a genetic basis. Children of a sleepwalker are six times more likely to be sleep walkers themselves than children of non-sleepwalkers (Hublin, et al., 1997).

Although no specific gene has been found to be responsible for insomnia, there have been several studies that have shown that insomnia can run in some families (e.g., Dauvilliers, et al., 2005; Drake, Scofield & Roth, 2008). There have also been studies that have shown that individuals who have identical twins who suffer from insomnia are more likely to also develop the disorder (e.g., Watson, Goldberg, Arguelles & Buchwald, 2006).

Your temperament is also influenced by genetics and is your characteristic way of responding emotionally and behaviorally to what occurs around you. A person's responses to situations are usually fairly stable over time and many of an individual's responses are thought to be innate. Some characteristic responses can even be observed in newborn babies! Although certain genes are believed to be involved, it is likely that temperament results from a complex interaction between many genes as well as environmental and developmental factors.

Your childhood experiences are also clearly likely to have predisposed you to certain sleep behaviors. For example, regular bedtimes as a child are likely to have reinforced particular beliefs about bedtime routines. Similarly, stressful childhood events around bedtime can result in conditioned responses to the experience of going to bed.

PRECIPITATING FACTORS

Sleep comes more easily than it returns.
- Victor Hugo, Les Misérables

Usually, periods of sleep loss are precipitated by life events which upset our normal routines or general sense of equilibrium. Insomnia usually begins during a time of stress, turmoil or upheaval. For example, you may have begun a new job, had a relationship breakdown, moved house or experienced significant inter-personal conflict. You may be predisposed to insomnia occurring under these circumstances because of one or more of the factors outlined in the previous section.

In any case, the result of these stressors is that your mind, and possibly also your body, has been working over-time, causing a temporary over-stimulation of your system. This over-stimulation can cause insomnia and can also cause disrupted eating patterns.

Some precipitating events happen over longer periods, making them more likely to have an impact on sleep quantity and quality. Some examples of precipitating events are:

A stressful life event;	Illness or surgery;
Interpersonal conflict;	Exposure to a traumatic event;
A period of uncertainty;	Relationship problems or divorce;
Job loss or change;	Work-related stress;
Personal loss;	Unemployment;
Ill health of a loved one;	Death of a loved one;
Upheaval in the home;	Legal difficulties;
Financial problems; and	Travel.

Often such insomnia is short-lived and you soon go back to your normal sleep patterns. However, in some instances, perpetuating factors come into play and the insomnia becomes more chronic or long lasting. While you may have little or no control over the precipitating factors that beset you, you can exert control over the perpetuating factors to prevent insomnia from developing into a longer-term problem.

PERPETUATING FACTORS

Generally speaking, insomnia is usually fundamentally caused by physiological or psychological hyper-arousal, meaning that your system is over-stimulated. This arousal may be caused by many factors or a combination of factors. Normally, arousal subsides over time, and our body returns to its normal state. However, many people unwittingly perpetuate their sleep problems by engaging in a whole range of behaviors and thoughts that they may think, at the time, will help solve the problem.

Some common perpetuating behaviors include paying attention to the sleep loss or trying to counteract the effects of it. Some common perpetuating thinking includes worrying about the sleep loss or engaging in negative 'self-talk' about it. Some examples of the latter are highlighted by the following quotes.

Sleeplessness is a desert without vegetation or inhabitants.

- Jessamyn West

The worst thing in the world is to try to sleep and not to.
                                        - F. Scott Fitzgerald

There is nothing so entirely desirable in all the world as a few hours'
oblivion.

                                        - Anne Reeve Aldrich

The language in these quotes typify something called 'cognitive distortion'. Some cognitive distortions are catastrophizing, all-or-nothing thinking, and focusing on the negative. We will get into more detail later about cognitive distortions and how they work.

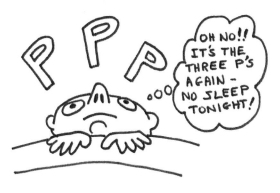

ACTIVITY

List below the predisposing, precipitating and perpetuating factors that may have contributed to you developing insomnia.

Predisposing factors:

_____
_____
_____
_____

Precipitating factors:

_____
_____
_____
_____

Perpetuating factors:

_____

_____

_____

_____

CONCLUSION

To summarize, chronic insomnia usually results from a combination of factors. Certain people are naturally predisposed to develop insomnia because of their temperament, genetics or other factors. Even without being predisposed to insomnia, a person can still develop chronic insomnia, so there is not much you can do about predisposing factors.

Precipitating factors, such as stressful events, often contribute to sleep loss in the first instance and cause a cycle of insomnia to start. You can learn to better control how you respond to precipitating factors in the future, but it is likely that if you are reading this book, the factors that precipitated your current sleep problems have happened in the past or recent past.

Perpetuating factors are those things that lead to insomnia becoming entrenched and make it seem like a problem that is out of control. Luckily, it is these factors that you can learn to address and by doing so, eliminate insomnia from your life.

REFERENCES

Bastien, C. H., Vallières, A. & Morin, C. M. (2001). Validation of the Insomnia Severity Index as an outcome measure for insomnia research. *Sleep Medicine, 2* (4), 297-307.

Centers for Disease Control & Prevention (2012). Short sleep duration among workers – United States, 2010. *Morbidity and Mortality Weekly Report, 61* (16), 281-285.

Chapman, D. P., Wheaton, A. G., Perry, G. S., Sturgis, S. L., Strine, T. W. & Croft, J. B. (2012). Household demographics and perceived insufficient sleep among US adults. *Journal of Community Health, 37*, 344-349.

Dauvilliers, Y., Morin, C., Cervena, K., Carlander, B., Touchon, J., Besset, A. & Billiard, M. (2005). Family studies in insomnia. *Journal of Psychosomatic Research.*, *58*(3), 271–278.

Drake, C. L., Scofield, H. & Roth, T. (2008). Vulnerability to insomnia: the role of familial aggregation. *Sleep Medicine*, *9* (3), 297-302.

Groeger, J. A., Zijlstra, F. R. H. & Dijk, D. J. (2004). Sleep quantity, sleep difficulties and their perceived consequences in a representative sample of some 2000 British adults. *Journal of Sleep Research*, *13*, 359-371.

Hublin, C., Kaprio, J., Partinen, M., Heikkila, K. & Koskenvuo, M. Prevalence and genetics of sleepwalking: A population-based twin study. *Neurology.*, *48*(1), 177–181.

Karlson, C. W., Gallagher, M. W., Olson, C. A. & Hamilton, N. A. (2013). Insomnia symptoms and well-being: Longitudinal follow-up. *Health Psychology*, *32* (3), 311-319.

Morin, C. M., Le Blanc, M., Bélanger, L., Ivers, H., Merette, C. & Savard, J. (2011). Prevalence of insomnia and its treatment in Canada. *Canadian Journal of Psychiatry*, *59* (6), 540-548.

Soldatos, C. R., Allaert, F. A., Ohta, T. & Dikeos, D. G. (2005). How do individuals sleep around the world? Results from a single-day survey in ten countries. *Sleep Medicine*, *6*, 5-13.

Watson, N. F., Goldberg, J., Arguelles, L. & Buchwald, D. (2006). Genetic and environmental influences on insomnia, daytime sleepiness, and obesity in twins. *Sleep*, *29* (5), 645-649.

Chapter 5

THE THINGS THAT HELP AND THOSE THAT DON'T

A flock of sheep that leisurely pass by,
One after one; the sound of rain, and bees
Murmuring; the fall of rivers, winds and seas,
Smooth fields, white sheets of water, and pure sky;
I have thought of all by turns, and yet do lie
Sleepless!

- William Wordsworth

INTRODUCTION

Of course, your ultimate goal is natural, good quality, refreshing sleep. With this in mind, there are many things that may help in the short, but not in the long, term. And there are things that may give you the *illusion* of having achieved a good night's sleep, when they haven't really been effective in providing you with good quality, sustainable, natural sleep. In this chapter, I will discuss some of the strategies that are helpful to people suffering from sleep loss and I will also explain why some of the things you may have tried are likely to have been less helpful.

SLEEP INDUCING SUBSTANCES

In most cases, people with insomnia turn to their primary health physician or general practitioner and in 95% of cases, these medical professionals prescribe medication to manage it (Charles, et al., 2009). Of these, about 80% of the medications prescribed tend to be in the benzodiazepine family (which includes Valium, Temazepam, Serepax, Mogadon and the like). The remaining 15% of insomnia sufferers are most often prescribed other sedatives or antidepressants. While pharmacological management of insomnia may be effective in the short term, it is often ineffective in the longer term and may also produce tolerance and dependence, and possibly other side-effects (Bartlett, 2014).

The other issue, of course, is that the sleep produced after sedative medications or substances is not a natural sleep and therefore, often does not contain all of the important properties of natural sleep in the normal amounts. For example, drinking a lot of alcohol can certainly make you "sleep", but it is not in fact good quality sleep. The normal stages of sleep are altered and it is likely that the sleep attained has not fulfilled its biological purposes for the body or brain. While sedative medication may provide you with improved sleep quantity, it often alters the normal sleep architecture.

In the short term, this may have the desired effect of making you feel more rested. However, it does not take very long for regular use of sedative medication to become habitual and to create a cycle of sedative-dependent sleep. This is because our very efficient bodies adapt to sedative medication in the same way as they adapt to alcohol. In other words, you soon develop a tolerance for them and in order to achieve the same effect, you then need to take a higher dose. Then you need an even higher dose, and so on.

If you try to then sleep without the medication, you will find that you experience *rebound insomnia*, which reinforces your belief that you need the medication to sleep (which by now, you do!) Thus, the dependence upon the sedative medication increases. Rebound insomnia is in fact a *withdrawal* symptom because most sedative medications are drugs of dependence. Although you may not tend to think of them in the same way as you think of heroin, nicotine and alcohol, you can become just as dependent upon them as with any type of drug that has an effect on your body that you desire or feel that you need.

I am not suggesting that you take yourself off any of your prescribed medications without first consulting with your physician. This is something that must be discussed with your physician and reduction of sedative medication should be done in a carefully controlled way under medical guidance.

What I am suggesting though, is that if you do decide (with your physician) to wean yourself off sedative medication, you will likely experience rebound insomnia and this is to be expected. However, this will be temporary and eventually you should be able to achieve a natural sleep if you are patient and persistent with the strategies outlined in this book.

TRYING HARDER

Many things - such as loving, going to sleep, or behaving unaffectedly - are done worst when we try hardest to do them.

\- C.S. Lewis

You may have heard of the story of people being instructed not to think about a pink elephant, which of course results in them not being able to stop thinking about a pink elephant! This story comes from experimental research conducted in 1987 by social psychologist, Daniel Wegner and his colleagues, who studied thought suppression by instructing research participants to avoid all thoughts of a white bear.

The researchers found that this resulted in the repeated return of a white bear in the thoughts of the participants. In fact they found that some participants even tended to think obsessively about white bears! If you apply this to sleep, the results are much the same. If you think a lot about insomnia, especially at bedtime, guess what happens? You suffer from insomnia! If you try not to think about insomnia, you also find yourself thinking about it more.

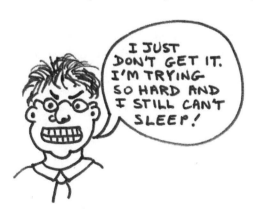

It's crazy how you can get yourself in a mess sometimes and not even be able to think about it with any sense and yet not be able to think about anything else.

– Stanley Kubrick

People who suffer from insomnia often make the mistake of trying harder to sleep, of forcing themselves to lie in their beds and close their eyes until sleep comes upon them. Unfortunately what tends to happen is that the very act of trying to get to sleep produces completely counterproductive results. It's kind of like trying to tell yourself to relax – it often doesn't work because it simply puts more pressure on you to achieve the desired result, which is not very conducive to relaxation.

This pressure increases psychological stress and arousal and this in turn wakes your body up more, in preparation for something that your unconscious mind sees as a threat. The more you tell yourself that insomnia leads to poor daytime functioning, the more real the threat feels and this heightens your inability to relax and sleep. Trying harder to sleep does not work – it is counter-productive and has the opposite effect to that which is desired.

WORRYING ABOUT NOT SLEEPING

The man who cannot sleep...refuses more or less consciously to entrust himself to the flow of things.

- Marguerite Yourcenar, Memoirs of Hadrian

Sometimes when you are laying in bed at night, you may find that you are feeling very tired, but you can't sleep because you are worrying about the possibility that you may have difficulty sleeping. You may be paying too much attention to this possibility and start planning what you might do if you can't get to sleep or what the next day will be like if you haven't slept well.

You might start to think about the things you need to be able to do the next day and the importance of being able to perform well. This heightened awareness of the threat of poor sleep is a type of hypervigilance. It is similar in some ways to the hypervigilance that soldiers in a war zone develop in order to be alert to potential dangers.

Unfortunately, hyperviligance increases your anxiety and can lead to exhaustion. It also increases your psychological arousal, which tends to make you more alert and less likely to fall asleep. You cannot afford to allow yourself to worry about sleep loss at all, but most especially you cannot afford to engage in this type of thinking when you are in the act of trying to fall asleep.

Similarly, if you wake during the night, this is not the time to become preoccupied with the possibility that you may not be able to return to sleep. It is better to think of something neutral or inconsequential, such as a pleasant holiday memory or a story you have enjoyed.

Worrying about not sleeping when you are trying to sleep is probably the most unhelpful thing you can do. This may seem very obvious to you now that I point it out, but it is surprising how many people who know this fact still engage in unhelpful worrying about loss of sleep.

WORRYING IN GENERAL

When I want to go to sleep, I must first get a whole menagerie of voices to shut up. You wouldn't believe what a racket they make in my room.

- Karl Kraus, translated from German by Harry Zohn

Sometimes when you have a lot of stress in your day, you may find that you lie in bed at night worrying about how to deal with the various concerns that have come up during that day or over an even longer period of time.

People who tend to worry a lot are certainly more vulnerable to insomnia, but worry is just a habit and, like any habit, it can be broken with practice and learning. You can neutralize it by replacing it with rational, more productive and helpful thinking patterns. Luckily, this can be learned.

In our busy society, sometimes the only time we get to be still with our thoughts is at night in bed. Also we have become accustomed to being able to switch things such as information gathering, lighting and entertainment on and off at will. The human brain cannot be switched on and off so easily.

We need to be more gentle with ourselves and allow our bodies and brains the opportunity to wind down and relax before bedtime, regardless of how this may shorten the time available to sleep. Our brain knows how to get the quantity and quality of sleep that it needs – we just have to learn to trust it.

TRYING TO CATCH UP ON LOST SLEEP

Of course, it is not uncommon for people suffering from insomnia, who are often tired, to try to catch up on *lost* sleep. This might involve napping, going to bed earlier or later than usual, sleeping in of a morning, or allowing yourself to nod off while watching TV.

That's fine if you sleep well at night, but if you have insomnia, the naps have to go, simple as that. The reason for this is that when naps are taken in the day, the body includes this nap time in its account of the total required amount of sleep and then you simply may not need as much sleep at night. If you are falling asleep while watching TV, take the hint that your body is giving you. Switch off the TV and go to bed.

There is between sleep and us something like a pact, a treaty with no secret clauses, and according to this convention it is agreed that, far from being a dangerous, bewitching force, sleep will become domesticated and serve as an instrument of our power to act.

- Maurice Blanchot

COMPENSATORY BEHAVIORS

When you feel that sleep loss is impacting on your ability to function on a day-to-day basis, it is only natural that you might try to compensate for this by adjusting your lifestyle to accommodate the consequences of sleeping poorly. While this seems natural and logical, it is actually counterproductive and feeds the problem. Unconsciously, you are saying to yourself: "This problem is bigger than I am. I will have to adapt my whole life around it."

Some examples of compensatory behaviors are:

- Changing your working hours to allow for inability to get out of bed by a certain time;
- Cancelling or shortening social engagements because you are too tired or think you will be too tired;
- Staying home or avoiding work because of a poor nights sleep;
- Rearranging your day to cope with the effects of sleep loss;
- Not taking on a project because you don't think you will be able to concentrate due to lack of sleep;
- Taking your own pillows on holiday with you; or

- Calculating how much sleep you've had overnight and then trying to work out how much sleep you'll need to make up for lost sleep.

In essence, you are not entrusting your own body to work it out and adapt. You are instead trying to control the situation and unconsciously giving power to the problem. Insomnia is a situation that is made worse by you trying to take control. You actually need to *relinquish* control. More importantly, you need to stop worrying about whether you can or can't control it.

It is similar, in many ways, to how agoraphobia develops. Usually, agoraphobia begins with a panic attack or anxious situation where the person feels a loss of control. Then they become anxious that this might occur again, and perhaps next time in a more public place. They begin to avoid such places and before long, they find themselves housebound. The avoidance feeds the anxiety and this leads to agoraphobia and isolation. Avoidance is actually the enemy but agoraphobics use avoidance to try to control the risk of panic attacks. Unwittingly, the more time they spend with the enemy (avoidance), the less likely they become to be able to overcome the problem.

Trying to take control and compensate does not relieve the anxiety. Nor does it resolve the insomnia. It merely perpetuates it. Engaging in behaviors that attempt to gain control of sleep patterns reinforces the belief that you can control something as biologically in-built as your heart beating. Sure, you can do things to relax and slow your heart rate down, but you cannot just stop or start your heart beating through sheer willpower. Similarly, sleep comes upon you when your body and brain is settled and when you need sleep.

ACTIVITY

List below some of the things you have been doing, in each of the above categories, that may have been unhelpful to getting a good, natural sleep.

Taking sedative substances:

_____

_____

_____

_____

Trying harder:

_____

_____

_____

_____

Worrying about not sleeping:

_____

_____

_____

_____

Worrying in general:

_____

_____

_____

_____

Trying to catch up on lost sleep:

_____

_____

_____

_____

Compensatory behaviors:

_____

_____

_____

_____

CONCLUSION

Sometimes we think we know better than our bodies do. We might think we need more sleep than we actually do. Remember, sleep is not one state. It is a complex mix of states and, at different times, your body may require more of one state than another. Luckily, you don't have to figure this out – your body does that for you. Relinquishing control of sleep and all its components, as counter-intuitive as this may feel, is actually a far better strategy than concerning yourself too much about how to get a certain amount of sleep or why you sleep less at certain times than others. The following chapters will explain exactly how to do that.

REFERENCES

Bartlett, D. (2014). Managing insomnia: What we've learnt in the last 10 years. *InPsych: The Bulletin of the Australian Psychological Society, 36* (2), 10-13.

Charles, J., Harrison, C. & Britt, H. (2009). Insomnia. *Australian Family Physician, 38* (5), 283.

Chapter 6

SPECIAL POPULATIONS

INTRODUCTION

Regardless of what your special circumstances may be, the information and strategies throughout this book can still be applied. However, there are certain populations that will benefit from some specific advice. There are many such populations and some require information and advice that goes beyond the scope of this book, so I will focus here on some populations that are relatively large. These are: long distance travellers; shift workers; women; older adults; adolescents; elite athletes; and parents of infants and small children.

LONG DISTANCE TRAVELLERS

When we travel across time zones and the bio-chemicals that our bodies are producing don't match up with the information coming in from our environment, we often feel the symptoms of jet lag. This affects everyone who travels long distances in short spaces of time. However, some of us adapt more quickly than others.

Another interesting factor is the effect of the direction of travel. If we travel across several time zones in a Westward direction, we tend to adapt more quickly than if we travel similar distances in an Eastward direction. Much research has been carried out to confirm this pattern and to try to uncover the reasons for the Eastward/Westward discrepancy.

Although this question has not yet been definitively answered, it has been suggested that Westward travel is consistent with an innate human tendency to gradually delay sleep onset as part of our natural circadian rhythm. You may have noticed that when you are on vacation and are completely unconstrained by commitments, you may tend to go to bed later and later each night?

Several studies have been conducted where research subjects spent several weeks in deep underground caves or laboratories where there were no stimuli, such as clocks, sunlight, outside sounds, radio or television, to indicate the time of day. They could turn on artificial lighting and engage in activities at will. The results showed that the subjects gradually went to sleep later and later until eventually the average length of their circadian day was 25 rather than 24 hours!

Nobody really knows why our bodies would have evolved this way. It doesn't seem to serve any purpose or relate to any time in the ancestral history of our species when this tendency may have been adaptive. Nevertheless, it is just one more mysterious aspect of sleep that gives us a small insight into how complex the sleep-wake cycle actually is.

And it helps to explain why we can't just switch sleep on or off at will or even, in an uncomplicated way, with medication. It's because so many different chemicals are involved and so many other unknown factors are also at play.

If you travel long distances on a regular basis, the crossing of time zones will have a similar effect on your body to that of shift work, and you will need to apply particular strategies for helping your body to adjust. When you are on short term, long distance trips, such as an overnight business trip, it is best if you can try to essentially keep to the time of your home country or base. Of course, it is likely that you will have to attend to commitments such as business meetings but the basic principle is that the adaptation you make should be as minimal as possible.

For example, if you travel from Los Angeles to London for an overnight business trip, there is an 8 hour time difference. Lets say that you leave at 8am and the journey takes 11 hours. Let's say that you had enough sleep the night before your trip so you don't sleep on the plane. You will arrive in London at around 3am (7pm LA time) London time. Let's say that you have a 9am (1am LA time) meeting and will be back on a plane at 5pm London time (9am LA time) to go back home to Los Angeles.

The best approach will be to go to bed at about 4am or 5am (8-9pm LA time), get up for your day of meetings (having had about 3 hours sleep), nap a little on the plane home, and then when you get home to LA at about 8pm, go to bed at around 9pm and get up the next morning at your usual time. Whilst in London, you should try to avoid morning sunlight as much as you can but expose yourself to sunlight in the afternoon.

The approach should be different for a longer journey. For example, if you travel from Sydney, Australia to Dubai (a 6 hour time difference) and plan to be there for 2 weeks, you need to work at adjusting your circadian cycle to the time zone in Dubai. This approach should begin in the week leading up to the journey. Dubai is 6 hours behind Sydney, so you would try to rise and go to bed an hour earlier for up to 6 days before the trip (obviously this has to work in with your work commitments and other obligations but the earlier you can manage, the better). So let's say that you have managed to go to bed at 8pm and get up at 4am by the time you leave. The most important part of this is making yourself get up at 4am because this will start to reset your circadian clock before you leave. This will make it easier for you to adapt when you reach Dubai.

Let's say that you are flying from Sydney at 9pm local time and the flight takes 13 hours. You should try to get to sleep as soon as you are able after you have boarded the plane. You will arrive in Dubai at 3am local time (10 am Sydney time). You should then try to sleep for a few hours but make sure you don't sleep any later than 8am local time, then get up and go out into the sunlight and spend all day being as active as possible. Then go to bed at 9pm or 10pm local time and try to operate on local time schedules for the duration of your trip.

When you return to Sydney, you will be likely to experience more trouble adapting because you are following a phase advance shift which is less in keeping with our natural tendency to follow a phase delay shift. However, the same principles will apply. Try to get closer to the patterns of your destination in the week leading up to travel; keep to the local time schedule when you reach your destination; and maintain sunlight exposure during the day, particularly in the morning.

SHIFT WORKERS

If you are a shift worker, you will also have to design some regularity around the shifts you are working. If you have a choice in the matter, the ideal shift rotation is to progress from an earlier starting time to a later one, rather than the other way around. For example, morning shifts, followed by a series of evening shifts, followed by a series of night shifts is going to be easier than night shifts followed by morning shifts. The worst kinds of shifts are those that swing backwards and forwards on a daily basis.

If you regularly work night shifts, you need to try to trick your body into turning everything in your 24-hour schedule around. Your daytime sleep period should be uninterrupted and treated in the same way that day workers treat nighttime. It is not unusual for night shift workers to try to get up after only a couple of hours sleep to attend to things like shopping or childcare and then try to sleep again before going back to work at night.

It is almost like the sleep of night-shift workers is regarded with less importance than sleep for regular workers. There is a misperception that night workers need less total sleep, which is absurd. When I was completing my PhD, I did night shifts in a hospital that finished at 7.30am. I would try to get to bed by 8.30am and sometimes I would get a phone call from a "friend" at midday. I would ask: "Don't you know I worked last night?" and would often get the response, "Yes, but it's midday – I thought you would have had enough sleep by now."

I know that this happens a lot to people who work night shifts. So take the phone off the hook or put it on silent. If you have to be available for family emergencies, make it very explicit that this is the only reason you can be called.

Essentially, you need to follow the same guidelines that I have outlined above for long distance travellers. If you are doing one night shift, is it not worth trying to change your circadian cycle around and then changing it back again in 24 hours. However, if you are going to be doing a week of night shifts, then you will have to make an adaptation.

So the adaptation is much like it would be if you were travelling to a country that has a 12-hour time difference from your base country. For example, if you are going to be working an 11pm to 7am shift for a week, your window for sleep is probably going to be from 8am to 10pm. Let's say that your usual bedtime is 10pm and you usually wake around 6am. The time difference for you, as it relates to sleeping is between 10 to 12 hours.

Your approach to adaptation should ideally begin in the week leading up to the night shifts. Your new sleep time is going to be 12 hours later than it is usually, so you would try to rise and go to bed an hour later for up to 6 days before the shift change (obviously this has to work in with your work commitments and other obligations but the later you can manage, the better).

So let's say that you have managed to go to bed at 1am and get up at 8am by the time you go on night shift. The most important part of this is making yourself get up at a later time because this will start to reset your circadian clock before you start night shifts. This will make it easier for you to adapt when you go onto the night shift.

After your first night shift, you should try to get to sleep as soon as you are able after your shift ends. Let's say that you manage to get to sleep at 8am. You should try to sleep for 7 to 8 hours and when you wake up, spend some time outside in the sunlight but not while the sun is setting, say around 4.30pm.Try to resist the urge to have a nap in the evening because this will confuse your system. You may be tired but the next day, you will probably sleep more solidly.

When you return to day shifts, the same principles will apply but it will be a lot easier to adapt because the light cues will be in synch with your sleep drive. Try to get a little closer to the patterns of your normal daytime routine towards the end of the time you are on night shift by rising and going to bed a little later; keep to your normal schedule once you are back in the land of the living; and maintain sunlight exposure during the day, particularly in the morning.

WOMEN

It is very common for women to report that their menstrual cycle affects their sleep patterns, usually three to six days prior to the onset of their period. Some women experience restless sleep, while others find it harder to get off to sleep or to stay asleep.

There are physical changes during the premenstrual phase caused by fluctuations in reproductive hormones and these changes have some measureable effects on sleep. For example, the amount of REM sleep is slightly reduced and body temperature is altered which also affects sleep.

Your approach to sleep around this premenstrual phase should be focused around keeping an even temperature during the night. You may need to wear lighter pajamas or have a cooler room temperature during this time of the month to make your sleep more comfortable. With REM sleep reduced, you may find that you wake up a little earlier than usual. There is no need to be concerned about this as it is quite natural.

Pregnancy is another time when sleep may be changed. Many women awaken more during pregnancy, especially during the third trimester when they may feel uncomfortable, experience sudden baby movements or have pressure on their bladder. Increased progesterone and estrogen may also reduce REM sleep. In addition, women are more likely to experience nasal congestion and snoring while pregnant, which can interrupt sleep.

Symptoms such as breast tenderness, heartburn, leg cramps, anxiety and vivid dreams also sometimes contribute to sleep loss in pregnancy. Women who have a tendency towards Restless Leg Syndrome (RLS) may experience an exacerbation of this during pregnancy or RLS may be experienced for the first time during pregnancy.

Your approach to sleep during pregnancy should be focused on the causes of your sleep disturbance. For example, if you are experiencing pressure on your bladder, you may have no option but to go to the toilet during the night. However, you don't need to put on bright lights when you get up and it is better to use a nightlight or subdued lamp so your brain doesn't get the idea that it is morning.

Restless Leg Syndrome during pregnancy is sometimes caused by gestational diabetes in which case, the cause can be treated. Similarly, RLS in pregnancy can be caused by iron deficiency, which can also be treated with iron supplements. However, some pregnant women experience the idiopathic type of RLS that has no known cause. For them, the treatment is symptomatic and remedies such as warm or cool showers or baths, heat packs, cold compresses, muscle stretching and avoidance of caffeine, alcohol and nicotine may be helpful.

Menopause is another time of major hormonal and psychological change when sleep can be disturbed. During the transition to menopause and during menopause itself, reduction of estrogen and progesterone can cause symptoms that interrupt sleep in some women. These include hot flashes, anxiety, depression and sleep-disordered breathing. Some women develop insomnia during this time, most likely perpetuated as a result of anxiety about sleep loss. As many as 61% of post-menopausal women report that they suffer from insomnia symptoms.

The focus of any approach to menopausal sleep loss needs to take into account the hormonal fluctuations that are occurring. The first step is to seek out a physician who specializes in this area to see what hormone replacement therapy may be safe in each individual case, if it is warranted. Depending upon the severity of the sleep loss, hypnotic medication may be helpful in the short term but some women find that this makes the hot flashes worse.

Where hot flashes are the main cause of the insomnia, care can be taken to keep cooler at night using such things as light clothing, fans and air conditioning. In addition, it can be helpful to avoid alcohol, nicotine, hot drinks and spicy foods, especially in the evenings. As with all types of insomnia, relaxation and exercise can also be helpful. Of course, all of the techniques in this book will also be useful in dealing with the perpetuating factors as well.

OLDER ADULTS

As we grow older, we spend less time in deep, slow-wave sleep and REM sleep, but more time in Stage 2 NREM sleep. In other words, our sleep is somewhat lighter as we become older and this is perfectly normal, particularly in older age. On average, adults need 7 ½ hours of sleep per night and the sleep requirement of individuals usually remains relatively stable into later adulthood.

However, sleep tends to become more fragmented, due to the changes in sleep architecture and older adults tend to report feeling less satisfied with the quality and quantity of their sleep. This is usually because of the fragmented, lighter sleep that is characteristic of the sleep of older adults. Sometimes, older people who experience these normal changes believe they are suffering from insomnia.

Even healthy older adults tend to achieve, on average, about 1 ½ hours less sleep than younger adults (Klerman & Dijk, 2008). In some cases, older individuals may experience insomnia or fragmented sleep because of sleep disorders such as sleep apnea or from physical ailments such as arthritic pain, respiratory or cardiac conditions. Depending on the symptoms and the full case history, the older person may require medical treatment, education, or insomnia treatment.

In general, all of the cognitive and behavioral approaches outlined in the coming chapters are very useful for older adults and research evidence strongly supports this. In addition, the causes of medical problems such as pain need to be addressed.

PARENTS OF INFANTS AND SMALL CHILDREN

We've all heard the term, "sleeping like a baby" and indeed babies tend to sleep a lot more than adults. Most teenagers have very different sleep patterns to those of younger children or adults. These differences are thought to be due to the differing needs of the brain and body as we grow and develop.

The sleep of newborns is irregular and interacts with their need to be fed at certain intervals. The amount of sleep required by newborns varies quite a lot and they may need anything from 10.5 hours to 18 hours per 24 hour cycle. They may sleep for anything from 5 minutes to several hours at a time and they may be light sleepers or extremely heavy sleepers. Generally, the sleep cycle of newborn babies is about 50 minutes in length, unlike the 70 to 100 minute cycle of adults.

Neonates also require a greater proportion of REM sleep, and REM sleep takes up as much as half of their overall sleep. In addition, the non-REM sleep of infants and children contains proportionately greater amounts of deep, slow wave sleep than that of adults. Growth Hormone is produced during this type of sleep, so slow wave sleep is thought to be important for physical growth and development.

As babies grow, they require less sleep and their sleep becomes more consolidated, so that by six months of age, many infants are sleeping through the greater part of the night in one sleep period. By this time, their sleep is comprised of about 30% REM and 70% non-REM sleep. By nine months of age, 70-80% of infants are sleeping through the night for about nine to twelve hours, and most are adapted to a cycle of sleeping more at night than during the day, with a couple of naps often still occurring during the day.

Parents of infants often complain of being sleep deprived and babies' crying at night is known to be the single factor that leads to the most sleep problems in new parents (Bayer, Hiscock, Hampton & Wake, 2007). Babies use crying to communicate a need, that of needing assistance and sometimes the assistance that is needed is to settle back to sleep. Parents often become confused about what need the baby is expressing at any given time. Is the baby hungry? Does the baby need a diaper change? Is the baby sick? Infants can't regulate their crying or problem solve, so they cry!

Parents who are fatigued as a result of sleep disturbance from infant waking and crying are significantly at risk of developing stress, anxiety and depression (Hiscock, Bayer, Hampton, Ukoumunne & Wake, 2008). Of course, they are also at risk of a whole lot of other problems, such as marital problems and even child abuse (El-Sheikh, Buckhalt, Mize & Acebo, 2006).

By 18 months of age, many children are napping only once per day, if at all, and sleeping 12 to 14 hours total across the 24 hour circadian day. Toddlers who nap too late in the day may experience difficulty settling at night. Also if they are very active or stimulated in the evening, or don't have regular bedtime and waking schedules, they may be unsettled at bedtime or during the night.

Pre-school age children usually sleep for between 11 and 13 hours per night and most stop napping by about 5 years of age. Children in this age group sometimes experience nighttime fears, nightmares and anxiety about being alone or in the dark at night. The occurrence of parasomnias, such as sleep walking, sleep talking and sleep terrors also tend to peak during this age period. This is probably because children of this age are still experiencing a proportionately greater amount of slow wave sleep than adults, especially in the first few hours of the night.

Once children are at school, they tend to need around 10 to 11 hours of sleep per night up until the age of about 12 years, and parents need to ensure that they get adequate sleep. This can be especially challenging as children become progressively more engaged in school, after-school, and entertainment activities, such as watching television and playing computer games.

The most common approach that is recommended to parents of infants and small children over six months of age who are presenting with behavioral insomnia is based on the idea that if the behavior (crying) is ignored, it will eventually stop or be *extinguished* because the infant will learn that it does not result in the desired result (the parents' presence). While variations on this approach, such as *controlled crying* have been virtually the only strategies available for decades, recent research has revealed that as many as 71% of parents won't use, or continue to use, these *extinction methods* (Blunden & Baills, 2013).

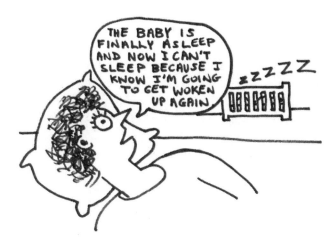

Alternative approaches called *cue-based methods* have been developed and are known to be successful and more acceptable to parents but they are less well known (Blunden, 2011, 2014). The cue-based approaches involve always calling out to the child, rocking and patting the child to sleep, introducing a comfort object and gradually reducing the rocking, then the patting, then the verbal comforting and encouraging the child to use the comfort object, with each step in the reduction process only introduced when the child's resistance and protest is also reduced.

ADOLESCENTS

On average, adolescents need around 9 ¼ hours sleep but for some, around 8 ½ hours is sufficient. During adolescence and early adulthood, our REM sleep requirement remains at least the same as for younger children but as a proportion of total sleep time, REM sleep increases slightly (Carskadon, 1982; Carskadon, Orav & Dement, 1983). Consistent with this, adolescents and young adults often get into a *phase delay* sleep pattern (Gradisar, Gardner, & Dohnt, 2011). This means that they tend to go to sleep later and get up later in the morning and this tendency is, at least to some extent, biologically determined and driven by the need for proportionately more REM sleep..

As a result, many adolescents do not get enough sleep because they have to be at school earlier than their natural wake time. Some high schools have even adopted later start and finish times to fit in better with the natural sleep-wake pattern of adolescents. On the whole, this has been found to improve academic performance, mood and attendance.

Of course, adolescents are also likely to be very busy with academic, social and work activities and in addition to that, they are also likely to be very engaged with electronic media, such as cell phones, computers, television and gaming, often within their bedrooms. All of this busyness and stimulation can be counter-productive when young people are attempting to get adequate quality sleep.

The most important aspects to assisting adolescents to obtain improved sleep are to reduce stimulating activities in the bedroom, such as computer games and television, and to encourage them to keep a regular sleeping schedule. That means that they need to go to bed at a similar time each night and more importantly, get up at roughly the same time each morning, even on weekends and during vacations.

If they don't do these things, they run the risk of developing *delayed sleep phase disorder*, which means that they go to bed and rise much later than others and start living the vampire lifestyle (i.e., sleep all day and wake all night). This is made worse by the fact that they then are less likely to experience sunlight at the crucial time of day for the setting of their circadian clocks, so they struggle to get back into a normal pattern. Adolescents can get sufficient sleep if they keep a regular sleep schedule and are disciplined about wake times, bed times and removing stimulation from the bedroom.

ELITE ATHLETES

You might imagine that elite athletes would be fantastic sleepers because they get lots of regular exercise, but this is not always the case. The amount of exercise that they do means that sometimes it is hard for them to relax and go to sleep. It adds to the problem that they are subject to the pressures of competing as well as stress and worry about always competing at their absolute best. Imagine if you carried the weight of your country's expectations of you to the Olympic Games, your big race was on in the morning and you couldn't sleep!

The other possibility is that your heats were on today and you are hyped up that you did well but now you have to get some sleep because the semi-finals are tomorrow. Excitement, international travel, strange beds and late night scheduling of sporting events all contribute to the problem of sleep loss in elite athletes. In addition, elite athletes often can't resort to using sedative medication because it may be banned within their sport.

Physical and mental stress each play a part in the sleep problems experienced by some elite athletes. This results in the stress hormone, cortisol, being released in response to this stress, exacerbating the situation and interfering with normal sleep architecture (Buckley & Schatzberg, 2005). Fear of poor performance adds to the pressure and stress, leading to sleep loss, which in turn leads to poor performance, causing the athlete to engage in a self-perpetuating cycle (McCloughan & Anderson, 2014).

All of the cognitive and behavioral approaches outlined in this book can be used by elite athletes, and if you are an elite athlete, it is best that you are familiar with, and practiced in, the strategies before you need to use them because it is probably too late to employ them by the time you are in the midst of high level competition.

CONCLUSION

If you belong to one of these, or other, special populations, you may need to be aware of the specific issues that apply to you when it comes to sleeping well and overcoming insomnia. Nevertheless, the same strategies essentially apply. Focusing on altering your sleep-related behaviors and thoughts so that they are more conducive to sleep is the most important thing to do. It is also helpful to modify your sleep hygiene and environment, taking into account some of the points raised in this chapter. Even if you don't have a sleep problem, you may find the tips in relation to long distance travel or shift work useful. The issues faced by elite athletes, I think, highlight the counter-productive effects of performance anxiety on sleep for all of us.

REFERENCES

Bayer, J. K., Hiscock, H., Hampton, A. & Wake, M. (2007). Sleep problems in young infants and maternal mental and physical health. *Journal of Pediatrics and Child Health, 43* (1-2), 66-73.

Blunden, S. (2011). Behavioral treatments to encourage solo sleeping in pre-school children: An alternative to controlled crying. *Journal of Child Health Care, 15* (2), 107-117.

Blunden, S. (2014). To cry or not to cry: The need for increased choice in behavioral sleep interventions for parents of infants. *InPsych: The Bulletin of the Australian Psychological Society, 36* (2), 16-17.

Blunden, S. & Baills, A. (2013). Treatment of Behavioral Sleep Problems: Asking the Parents. *Journal of Sleep Disorders: Treatment and Care, 2*(2), 1-7.

Buckley, T. & Schatzberg, Z. (2005). On the interactions of the hypothalamic-pituitary adrenal (HPA) axis and sleep: normal HPA axis activity and circadian rhythm, exemplary sleep disorders. *Journal of Clinical Endocrinology and Metabolism, 90* (5), 3106-3114.

Carskadon, M. A. (1982). The second decade. In C. Guilleminault (Ed.), *Sleeping and Waking Disorders: Indications and Techniques* (99-125). Menlo Park, CA: Addison-Wesley.

Carskadon, M. A., Orav, E. J. & Dement, W. C. (1983). Evolution of sleep and daytime sleepiness in adolescents. In C. Guilleminault & E. Lugaresi

(Eds.), *Sleep/Wake Disorders: Natural History, Epidemiology, and Long-Term Evolution*, (201-216). New York, NY: Raven Press.

El-Sheikh, M., Buckhalt, J. A., Mize, J. & Acebo, C. (2006). Marital conflict and disruption of children's sleep. *Child Development, 77* (1), 31-43.

Gradisar, M., Gardner, G. & Dohnt, H. (2011). Recent worldwide sleep patterns and problems during adolescence: A review and meta-analysis of age, region and sleep. *Sleep Medicine, 12*, 110-118.

Hiscock, H., Bayer, J. K., Hampton, A., Ukoumunne, O. C. & Wake, M. (2008). Long-term mother and child mental health effects of a population-based infant sleep intervention:cluster-randomized, controlled trial. *Pediatrics, 122* (3), e621-e627.

Klerman, E. B. & Dijk, D-J. (2008). Age-related reduction in the maximal capacity for sleep - implications for insomnia. *Current Biology, 18* (15), 1118-1123.

McCloughan, L. & Anderson, R. (2014). Disordered sleep in elite athletes – possible solutions. *InPsych: The Bulletin of the Australian Psychological Society, 36* (2), 18-19.

Chapter 7

A COMPREHENSIVE APPROACH

It always seems impossible until it's done.

- Nelson Mandela

INTRODUCTION

In this chapter, I will explain how hyper-arousal, in its many forms, is the main culprit when it comes to insomnia. I will also describe a little about the biochemistry of sleep, and explain the various roles of many different, naturally produced bio-chemicals in relation to sleep. I will show you why we can't easily turn sleep on or off and outline why an emphasis on behavior and thinking is the best way to tackle insomnia. I will list the different non-pharmacological therapies that are commonly used for insomnia and show how they are rated according to clinical evidence regarding patient outcomes.

IT WON'T HAPPEN OVERNIGHT, SO BE PATIENT!

It's important to keep in mind when using the strategies outlined in this book that some of the techniques discussed may not have an immediate effect on your sleep. Sometimes it may take a few days, weeks or months of making a change to your schedule, thought patterns and behaviors before your body adjusts. This is normal, and you should not give up on making a change if it doesn't immediately improve your sleep.

It is likely that your sleep problems have developed over a long period of time. They may also take a long period of time to become resolved. I'm guessing that what you've been doing so far hasn't worked very well, so you need to devote yourself to the strategies in this book whole-heartedly, patiently and consistently over a long period of time for them to work for you.

THE ROLE OF HYPER-AROUSAL

In almost all cases, insomnia is caused by overall hyper-arousal, which may be physical, psychological or both. Hyper-arousal can be due to a number of different causes. For example, people who take stimulants are in a state of physical hyper-arousal. Similarly, people who have just been through a frightening ordeal are likely to be in a state of physical and psychological arousal. The majority of people with chronic insomnia don't take stimulants. Nor have most of them just experienced a frightening ordeal. So why can't they sleep?

Hyper-arousal is caused and perpetuated by many factors, many of which were listed in Chapter 4. Hyper-arousal is not just a factor at bedtime – it is a factor all day and night. For example, if you work in a high-powered job and you never give yourself the opportunity to relax, you are probably in a constant state of physical and psychological hyper-arousal. This is not only problematic for your sleep, but for your health in general.

Most of the techniques outlined in this handbook are designed around reducing hyper-arousal. Essentially, when you know how to do this and about how to stop engaging in counter-productive behaviors and thinking, you will know how to beat insomnia.

When we are very involved in a physical activity such as running, our bodies produce a number of chemicals to help us perform this activity. These chemicals are designed for a particular purpose and they need to be out of our systems for our bodies to engage in opposite purposes like relaxing and sleeping. Physical activities, such as running are excellent for using up chemicals such as adrenalin.

When we are engrossed in a mental activity such as problem solving or negotiating a new relationship or business deal, our bodies produce chemicals and hormones that are designed for those particular purposes. Again, these neuro-substances need to be out of our bodies when we are trying to relax and sleep.

Unlike physical activity, mental activity doesn't use these chemicals up in such a direct way. This is because, when we are awake, we are constantly engaged in some sort of mental activity and our bodies can't always detect the fine differences between mental activities that require a lot of concentration and those that don't. So these chemicals leave our system more slowly.

Physical exercise can sometimes help with this because, especially if it requires significant effort, it stops us from being able to concentrate so hard. Also, some of the chemicals that are used and produced during exercise, such as adrenaline, are also produced in response to some mental activities.

Hyper-arousal is caused by the way we think and also by the way that we act. In addition, elements of our environment can contribute to hyper-arousal. Can you imagine trying to sleep on the hard floor of a noisy casino?

The approach outlined in this handbook focuses on addressing hyper-arousal across the three spheres of thinking, behavior and the environment. If you were to focus on just one of these spheres, your insomnia would probably continue. You have to take a comprehensive approach in order to address your insomnia, once and for all.

THE BIOCHEMISTRY OF SLEEP

Fasten your seatbelts. It's going to be a bumpy night.
                                                    – Joseph L. Mankiewicz

You don't really need to know about the biochemistry of sleep to be able to address your insomnia, but I'll discuss it here for those who might be interested. Skip over it if you're not all that fascinated by the scientific aspects of sleep. I guess the point of this is to show you that sleep is really quite a complicated phenomenon and also to explain why it is not a simple matter to turn it on and off.

Arousal of the cortex of the brain occurs via two pathways of nerve tracts. One involves the thalamus and one involves the hypothalamus and basal forebrain. Various clusters of cells at the terminals of these tracts produce, when turned on, a range of neuro-chemicals that have an effect on wakefulness and sleepiness.

There are many, many bio-chemicals involved in the regulation of the sleep-wake cycle and this is why no pharmaceutical company has yet come up with a drug to cleanly induce sleep or wakefulness without side effects.

Believe me; they continue to work hard at it though! The bio-chemicals that regulate, or are regulated by, sleep, include:

- Glutamate (produces arousal of the whole cerebral cortex)
- Histamine (produces arousal of the whole cerebral cortex)
- Orexin or hypocretin (produces arousal of the whole cerebral cortex)
- Acetylcholine (contributes to arousal of the cerebral cortex)
- Seratonin (influences the cortex to modulate sleep and waking)
- Noradrenaline (influences the cortex to modulate sleep and waking)
- Norepinephrine (along with serotonin, indirectly regulates REM sleep by inhibiting the cells that produce acetylcholine)
- Dopamine (influences the cortex to modulate sleep and waking)
- Gamma-aminobutyric acid (GABA) (inhibits the cells that produce histamine, thus mediating arousal of the cerebral cortex; GABA is sometimes referred to as the brain's "dimmer switch")
- Growth hormone releasing hormone (GHRH) (activates the cells that are receptive to GABA to inhibit arousal of key parts of the brain involved in sleep)
- Adenosine (modulates arousal by inhibiting the cells that produce acetylcholine)
- Melatonin (produced by the pineal gland in response to low light signals as it gets dark that are received by two tiny clusters of cells called the suprachiasmatic nuclei near the optic nerve)
- Tryptophan (a precursor amino acid, which is converted in the brain to serotonin, which is then made into melatonin by the pineal gland)
- Human growth hormone (production of this hormone surges during the first three hours of sleep)
- Cortisol (secreted during the last part of sleep, it reaches its peak upon awakening)
- Prolactin (increases 60-90 minutes after sleep onset, peaking in the early morning hours)

My sincere apologies to any neuro-chemicals or hormones that I have missed out!!! I guess my point here is that several parts of the brain are involved and many natural chemicals produced by the body are involved in whether we are awake or asleep at any given time. Importantly, they all become potentially involved when we become physically or psychologically hyper-aroused.

In addition to all the natural hormones and neuro-chemicals that influence sleep and wakefulness, there are many more that are produced or inhibited depending upon what point in the sleep-wake cycle we are in at any given moment. For example, our digestive system periodically releases certain chemicals to tell us we are hungry during wakefulness but these are suppressed during sleep. This is why we get hungry at odd times when we are sleep deprived or jet lagged.

THE ELUSIVE ON/OFF SWITCH

Some researchers have suggested that when we understand enough about how our circadian clock works, we ought be able to override it, for example, with drugs that could turn sleep on and off pharmacologically. When the contraceptive pill was introduced in the 1960s, people got the idea that almost any natural biological function could be altered and artificially regulated. While the contraceptive pill is successful in preventing pregnancy, it does not, for the most part, have a reliable impact on the natural sex drive. The drive for sleep is also a strong biological drive, and altering a fundamental human drive is much more complicated.

Not to be deterred, many drug companies around the world are striving to develop drugs that could turn sleep on and off, without dangerous side effects. Think how much more we could get done if we only needed one to two hours of sleep per night! Amphetamines and other stimulants have been used by people for decades to stay awake, but they tend to result in unpleasant side effects including a "crash" after they wear off, where the user needs to sleep and recover.

Then in the mid-1990s, along came a new class of *vigilance promoting drug* called *eugeroics* (Greek for good arousal) that promoted wakefulness without the euphoria, addictiveness and nasty after-effects of stimulants. The first of these drugs to become widely available has been Modafinil, which was originally developed for sufferers of a rare disorder called narcolepsy. This devastating REM sleep disorder is characterized by sudden bouts of REM sleep that intrude on wakefulness (cataplexy), daytime sleepiness and intrusion of dreams into waking life. Narcoleptics had traditionally been prescribed amphetamines to combat daytime sleepiness, so Modafinil, when in came along, represented a huge improvement in the treatment of narcolepsy.

Before long, Modafinil, which could produce 48 hours or so of uninterrupted alertness, was being prescribed "off label" for anything from shift work to cocaine dependence, and there have been numerous court cases about whether or not it was being promoted for reasonable purposes. Not surprisingly, it has now become somewhat of a lifestyle drug, with surprisingly high numbers of college students obtaining and using the drug to stay awake and study, giving them a purported edge over other students.

Still other drugs are being developed to attempt to condense sleep into a shorter period of "super sleep". As you can imagine, the military of some nations are very interested in such substances and the prospect of using them to enhance the capacity of military personnel in combat.

While the search goes on for pharmacological on and off switches for sleep and waking, most of us continue to seek and enjoy good quality natural sleep. Intuitively, we know that artificial sleep inducers are likely to come at a cost and that such costs may not be apparent until many years later.

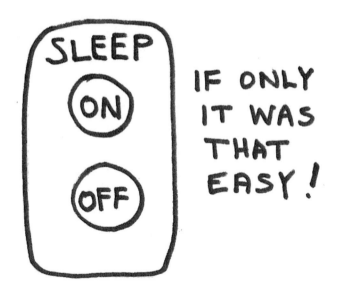

BEHAVIOR, THINKING AND ENVIRONMENT ARE WHAT IT'S ALL ABOUT

Cognitive Behavioral Therapy (CBT) has been around in various forms since the 1950s and there are more studies to show that it is effective for a whole range of problems than for any other kind of therapy. Most commonly,

CBT is used to help people with anxiety or depression, but it is also used for a wide range of other problems. Since the early 2000s, CBT that focuses on helping people with insomnia (CBT-i) has been developed and its effectiveness has been measured and there is now strong evidence that it is highly effective.

According to many contemporary studies, randomized controlled trials and professional sleep bodies, CBT-i is now considered the best first line treatment for chronic insomnia (Bartlett, 2014; Morgenthaler, et al., 2006; Morin, et al., 2006; Schutte-Rodin, et al., 2008). It has also been shown to be more effective than hypnotic medication (Siversten, et al., 2006). There are a range of different types of CBT-i, varying according to their emphasis on, and approaches to, thinking or cognition and behavior.

Specific types of CBT-i include the following. I have indicated beside each one the level of recommendation that has been assigned to each therapy by the Standards of Practice Committee of the American Academy of Sleep Medicine (Morgenthaler, et al., 2006). *Standard recommendation* represents the highest level of recommendation and this means that there is a high degree of clinical certainty that the therapy is effective and that there is very good clinical research evidence for its use. *Guideline recommendation* is the second highest level of recommendation, which reflects a moderate degree of clinical certainty. *Option recommendation* means that no recommendation can be made at this time as there is inconclusive evidence for its clinical use.

- Stimulus control therapy (Standard);
- Sleep restriction or bed restriction (Guideline);
- Psychological and behavioral interventions (Standard);
- CBT (Standard);
- Paradoxical intention (Guideline);
- Biofeedback (Guideline);
- Sleep hygiene education (Option);
- Relaxation training (Standard); and
- Imagery training (Option).

ACTIVITY

List below some of the things you have already tried in an effort to get better sleep. Then place a tick beside those that you found helpful. Place two ticks beside those that were helpful over a long period, such as a year.

_____

_____

_____

_____

_____

_____

_____

_____

CONCLUSION

The comprehensive approach outlined in this handbook utilizes CBT, cognitive therapy, stimulus control therapy, and sleep hygiene education. Relaxation training is certainly something, like regular exercise, that is very useful in reducing physiological arousal and I will include these approaches under sleep hygiene education. I will briefly touch on, and explain some of the other approaches as well. Unfortunately, we have become an impatient society and we generally expect to be able to access everything quickly, which is why many people expect their physicians to provide them with pills that work as on or off switches. This is not realistic and our bodies are much too complicated to be able to be dealt with that way. There are all sorts of fail-safe mechanisms built into our bodies, such as tolerance, so that even if a pill works for a while, we become tolerant to its effects. The strategies outlined in this book work with our brains and bodies in ways that are completely natural and this is why they work in the longer term.

REFERENCES

Bartlett, D. (2014). Managing insomnia: What we've learnt in the last 10 years. *InPsych: The Bulletin of the Australian Psychological Society, 36* (2), 10-13.

Morgenthaler, T., Kramer, M., Alessi, C., Friedman, L., Boehlecke, B., Brown, T., Coleman, J., Kapur, V., Lee-Chiong, T., Owens, J., Pancer, J. & Swick, T. (2006). Practice parameters for the psychological and behavioral treatment of insomnia: An update. An American Academy of Sleep Medicine Report. *Sleep, 29* (11), 1415-1419.

Morin, C. M., Le Blanc, M, Daley, M., Gregoire, J. P. & Merette, C. (2006). Epidemiology of insomnia: prevalence, self-help treatments, consultations, and determinants of help-seeking behaviors. *Sleep Medicine, 7,* 123-130.

Schutte-Rodin, S., Broch, L., Buysse, D., Dorsey, C. & Sateia, M. (2008). Clinical guideline for the evaluation and management of chronic insomnia in adults. *Journal of Clinical Sleep Medicine, 4* (5), 487-504.

Siversten, B., Omvik, S., Pallesen, S., Bjorvatn, B., Havik, O. E., Kvale, G., Nielsen, G. H. & Nordhus, I. H. (2006). Cognitive behavioral therapy vs zopiclone for treatment of chronic primary insomnia in older adults: a randomized controlled trial. *Journal of the American Medical Association, 295* (24), 2851-2858.

Chapter 8

CHANGING YOUR BEHAVIOUR

It is better to light one candle than to curse the darkness.
— James Keller

INTRODUCTION

The only way to improve your sleep and overcome insomnia is to focus on changing the way you think and also the way that you behave. This chapter is focused on changing your behavior, with a particular focus on sleep hygiene and a strategy called stimulus control. When you begin to master these strategies, you will gain confidence into your ability to achieve satisfying sleep.

WHICH ARE THE MOST EFFECTIVE BEHAVIORAL STRATEGIES?

Stimulus control therapy is classified by the Standards of Practice Committee of the American Academy of Sleep Medicine at the highest level of recommended treatment for insomnia, which means there is a very high level of clinical certainty that it is effective (Morgenthaler, et al., 2006).

The same level of recommendation has been given to cognitive behavioral therapy, so we will be utilizing that in this, and the next, chapter. There is insufficient evidence regarding the use of sleep hygiene alone, but I have found that education about sleep hygiene is helpful as an adjunct to stimulus control therapy. It is all fairly simple and straightforward and you should find it relatively easy to follow the strategies that are outlined below.

It is important to note however, that changing behavior alone will not resolve the insomnia. The thinking aspect must be tackled as well. It is only through a combination of changing thinking and behavior that insomnia can be overcome. You will also find as you use the approaches below that thinking and behavior are linked and addressing one will often help with working on the other.

SLEEP HYGIENE

You may have been told by your doctor or by a friend that you need to practice better *sleep hygiene*. What is sleep hygiene? It sounds like some kind of bedtime cleaning ritual! I don't know where the term came from originally but what sleep hygiene amounts to is the kinds of things your grandmother may have suggested to help you get a good night's sleep. And grandma wasn't too far off the mark!

Most sleep hygiene strategies relate to ensuring your environment is conducive to sleep but also to you doing things like taking a warm bath and reducing stimulation before bedtime. Sleep hygiene is certainly helpful but it doesn't work on its own – you have to also address your thinking and behaviors in relation to sleep.

Sleep hygiene is also all about conditioning your mind to prepare for sleep at the right time of day through regular and repetitive practices. If you consistently perform the same tasks and rituals before going to bed, your brain is likely to start to associate these activities with bed, sleep and tiredness.

By keeping a bedtime ritual that is similar from night to night, you will help to prepare your body and your brain for sleep. Similarly, when you wake up during the night, repeating some of these activities should make it easier for you to return to sleep.

Here are some examples of bedtime rituals you could try:

- Go to bed and meditate for 5 minutes, focusing entirely and completely on your breathing;
- An hour before bed, have a warm shower or bath and get changed into your pajamas or nightdress;
- After your shower or bath, turn off any overhead lights and use table lamps instead;

- Twenty minutes before bedtime, have a small cup of herbal tea;
- Undertake your standard pre-bedtime cleansing routine, e.g., brush your teeth, wash your face;
- Read for 15 minutes on the couch.

These rituals can be adapted to include the things you find very relaxing, and to exclude things you think will agitate or stimulate you. Take the opportunity to be a bit creative with your rituals, and consider which activities are most likely to calm your body down for sleep.

PREPARING YOUR BODY FOR SLEEP

One reason some people have problems getting to sleep is that their body doesn't actually realize when they're trying to get to sleep. In some ways, your body has a mind of its own. This is related to an unconscious process that psychologists call the *power of association*. When you spend long periods in bed lying awake, your brain unconsciously starts to associate being in bed with being awake.

This can begin to work against you in your efforts to get to sleep. You should try to avoid reading, watching TV, reading emails, doing internet searches or eating when in bed, as these are "awake-time" activities. You want to train your body into thinking it should be asleep soon after you get into bed.

MAINTAINING REGULAR SLEEP HABITS

When you have been experiencing insomnia for a period of time, it is likely that your bedtimes and wake times vary a lot. But as you get used to using the different techniques you will read about here, you will be able to identify an approximate time when you are best able to put yourself to bed. Then working back from this time, you will be able to identify the hours in which it is best not to engage in stimulating activities.

Similarly, you will in due course identify a time when you seem to get up more easily and habitually. You may need to use bright light early in the morning (the easiest way is by opening the curtains for morning sun) in order to help your body adjust to the same regular waking time each day. In keeping this morning light ritual, you are likely to develop a natural routine of waking up at a regular time.

If your sleep patterns are seriously out of alignment, the most important thing to focus on is the time of day that you wake up in the morning. Set a regular time for rising, set your alarm, and get up at that time, no matter what kind of night you have had, even if you haven't slept at all. If you keep doing this every day, your body will eventually get the message.

To reset your circadian clock, the most important thing to do is to rise from bed at the same time each morning regardless of the previous night's sleep and regardless of what time you went to bed. The next most important thing to do is to experience morning light and reduce exposure to bright light in the evening. This will ensure that your body is releasing melatonin at the right time, which also helps reset your circadian rhythm.

You need to be consistent – it's like doing behavior modification on yourself. The same regular rising time will reinforce the change in your behavior and it will become a pattern that you will get used to.

RELAXATION TRAINING

You may find it difficult to find time to learn about or practice relaxation training but the reality is that it is easy and quick to learn and you only need to devote as little as 15 minutes per day to practicing it. There are loads of apps and CDs that will guide you through various types of relaxation and it is simply a matter of finding the type that suits you best.

Some people like to do progressive muscle relaxation and others prefer yoga-based relaxation, while others find relaxation involving guided imagery the most effective. My advice is to try a few different types out and see what works for you. You will find some useful websites, apps and resources in Appendix 1 that will lead you to relaxation strategies that you can try.

Practicing some form of relaxation or meditation for as little as 15 minutes per day can reduce your overall levels of arousal and this may help reduce your sleep loss. Usually insomnia is caused by a combination of factors and addressing insomnia is likewise usually resolved by a combination of approaches. The main focus is reducing arousal and relaxation, and practiced regularly, relaxation will certainly help you to achieve that.

PRACTICING RELAXATION BEFORE BEDTIME

Although sleep is a natural process that your body goes through every day, it is still necessary for you to prepare for sleep in order to obtain maximum benefit from it. The more relaxed you are before going to bed, the easier it will be for you to get to sleep. This can often be difficult if you have a lot of hustle and bustle going on in the last few hours of the day.

Taking just 15 or more minutes to relax before you go to bed can make it easier to get to sleep. Try doing some light reading, listening to quiet music, or meditating. Any activity that relaxes you should help your body to prepare for the sleep cycle.

This also means that if you can, you should try to avoid any activities that are exciting or stressful (such as involved telephone conversations, cleaning, watching thrillers on TV, or going over your finances) in the last couple of hours of the day. If you have daily commitments that tend to get you anxious or frustrated, try to schedule these activities for earlier in the day, so that they don't interfere with your sleep.

CLOCK OFF

To sleep is an act of faith.

- Barbara G. Harrison

If you are continually glancing at the clock during the night, this is more likely to make you worry about the fact that you aren't in a state of continual sleep, and ironically, this worry may keep you awake! Clock-watching is not allowed, so you need to either remove all clocks (and this includes cell phones) from your bedroom, or place them completely out of sight (e.g., just under your bed). If you do decide that you need to keep the clock or cell phone in the bedroom (e.g., for the purposes of waking to an alarm), make sure you don't check it at all during the night. Having an alarm clock by the bed can sometimes be more stressful than helpful.

If you need an alarm clock to wake you in the morning, have it low down or turned away from you so that the time is not visible to you when you are in bed. Similarly, don't check the time on your cell phone or computer if you wake up during the night. It is better to not pay too much attention to when or whether you wake during the night.

The other problem with electronic devices in the bedroom is that they often give off light through small LED charger lights. It is best not to have any unnecessary lights shining in your bedroom at night.

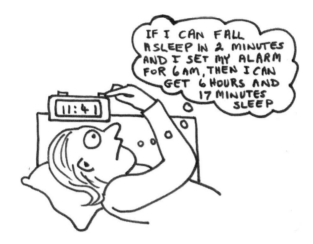

EXERCISE

Exercise stimulates your nervous system and then produces a natural tiredness. Most people who exercise regularly find it beneficial to their health generally and it tends to be helpful as part of a combination of approaches in helping people with insomnia. However, you should avoid exercising directly before bedtime, as the resulting stimulation may spill over into the time period when you need to be winding down for sleep.

As it gets closer to bedtime, your body temperature naturally begins to fall slightly, helping to signal to your body that it is time to get sleepy. Exercise raises your body temperature and it stays up for up to 5 hours, so if you have a sleep problem, it is better to avoid exercise after 5pm. Exercising in the late afternoon is ideal because when the body temperature does eventually drop down, this reinforces the natural fall in temperature in the later evening.

If you exercise in the morning, it is even better if you combine it with exposure to sunlight as both of these things help to re-set your circadian clock if it is out of kilter. If you live in a place where you don't have access to natural sunlight in the morning, you can purchase specialized artificial light boxes. There is more information about these in Chapter 10.

Regular exercise is also known to help with general stress and muscle tension, so it is indirectly helpful in relaxing at night in preparation for sleep. At least twenty minutes of cardiovascular exercise three or four times per week is helpful in this regard and it has also been shown to improve mood.

NO MORE NAPS!

Sorry! Every human body needs a particular and individual amount of sleep in each daily 24-hour circadian cycle. When this amount of sleep has been met, it can be difficult for you to fall asleep, as your body has energy that it wants to consume. Some people like to take naps in the day, and this practice can sometimes increase with age.

Some research has been carried out on the type of sleep that occurs when people nap, and the results were quite interesting. As you now know, we tend to get more deep, slow-wave sleep in the first half of the night and more REM sleep in the second half of the night. Naps seem to reflect this characteristic of nightly sleep. If you nap in the morning, your nap is more likely to contain REM sleep and if you nap in the afternoon, the nap is more likely to contain slow wave sleep.

Of course, this is largely dependent on your sleep debt and also how long you nap for. If the nap is less than 20 minutes long, you are unlikely to get past light Stage 2 sleep. If it is longer, you may drift into deep sleep or REM sleep. This is why, if you have a long nap, you sometimes wake feeling quite groggy and unrefreshed. This is called *sleep inertia* and this is the reason that shift workers who are able to take a sleep break during their shift are better to limit these breaks to half an hour or less.

By stopping taking naps, you will find it easier to fall asleep at a reasonable hour in the mid to late evening. People who don't nap are also less likely to wake up very early in the morning or have trouble staying asleep during the night. In short, if you are not sleeping well at night, napping can make matters worse because the body's need for sleep at night is reduced.

If you are used to taking naps in the day, you may initially find that this leaves you feeling unusually tired for a few days. When this tiredness sets in, try sitting in brighter light (preferably natural sunlight) and undertaking an engaging activity, such as doing some stimulating work, housework, having a discussion with a friend or work colleague, calling someone on the telephone or going for a walk outside for five to ten minutes.

BIOFEEDBACK

Biofeedback therapy can only be done with a specialist therapist who has the appropriate equipment. Biofeedback is used to train you to recognise and lower your level of physiological arousal, usually by watching a monitor that tells you about indicators of physical measures, such as heart rate, breathing rate, and brain waves (via electroencephalograph or EEG).

Biofeedback can be quite useful and effective but can also be expensive and inconvenient compared to approaches that can be employed at home without the direct involvement of equipment or a therapist. In addition, it will not work on its own as the thinking (cognition) aspect of insomnia can still intrude and interfere, even if the person knows how to regulate their arousal levels.

Biofeedback also does not have as much research evidence for its effectiveness as CBT-i or Stimulus Control. For this reason, it is only recommended if you have already tried these other therapies and wish to add another skill to your toolkit.

SLEEP RESTRICTION OR BED RESTRICTION

Fatigue is the best pillow.

- Benjamin Franklin

Sleep restriction works on the principle that time in bed will become more efficient in being taken up with sleep if it is restricted. This idea is based on the fact that when people are completely deprived of sleep for a few nights, they tend to sleep very solidly afterwards. Sleep restriction enhances the sleep drive by restricting the window of opportunity for sleep.

Sleep restriction works like this:

1. The person keeps a sleep diary for a couple of weeks.
2. The average total nightly sleep time is worked out from the sleep diary (lets say it is 5 hours).
3. The person only allows themselves to be in bed for this average amount of time (in our example, 5 hours) for one week, by setting strict bedtimes and waking times.
4. Usually by the end of the week, the person is sleeping for at least 85% of the total time spent in bed (in our example, at least 4 ¼ hours).

5. If this goal has been achieved, the person can allow themselves 15-20 minutes more sleep per night for the following week (in our example, if the person is sleeping 4 ¼ -5 hours, they may now stay in bed for 5 ¼ hours to 5 hours and 20 minutes).
6. If 85% or more sleep efficiency has been achieved by the end of the second week, total time in bed can again be increased by another 15-20 minutes.
7. Total time in bed continues to be increased in this way every week until the person is achieving a full night of restorative sleep.

In practice, it can be quite difficult to self-enforce the sleep restriction regime, although it is usually very effective in consolidating sleep and improving continuity of sleep. The person may also be quite sleepy in the daytime and there may be concerns about safety with driving and the like.

It may be difficult for the person to prevent themselves from napping or having micro-sleeps because the sleep drive is so powerful. For these reasons, unless the person is on vacation and can be supervised in the process by a spouse, partner or friend, I prefer to suggest the stimulus control technique rather than the sleep restriction technique.

STIMULUS CONTROL

If you can't sleep, then get up and do something instead of lying there worrying. It's the worry that gets you, not the lack of sleep.
                                                            - Dale Carnegie

The rationale behind stimulus control is based on *classical conditioning theory*. People who have experienced chronic insomnia over a period of time can come to associate the bed, and even the bedroom, with the frustration and worry of not sleeping. Stimulus control aims to break or extinguish this association. The idea is that you instead begin to clearly associate the bed with the positive experience of sleeping, so that being in the bed unconsciously signals to your brain that it is time for sleep. The power of association and conditioning is thought to be very strong in relation to insomnia.

The number one rule with stimulus control is to only go to bed when sleepy. So you need to pay attention to when you do feel sleepy. There are two natural dips in our daily circadian rhythm: One occurs about 8 hours after we wake up in the morning (so this is usually mid-afternoon) and the other stronger dip occurs in the mid to late evening when we usually go to bed.

I'm sure you have had that experience where you keep falling asleep during the evening and fight it because you are trying to get something done, sit through a late meeting or watch a television program, or perhaps because you think it is too early to go to bed. Ironically, you later wake right up and can't get to sleep when you finally do go to bed. This is because you have effectively missed the natural dip in your cycle and not responded to the sleepy signals your body was trying to send to you earlier in the evening.

So part of stimulus control is to try to schedule your obligations, social life and working patterns so that you can go to bed in the evening when you do feel sleepy, rather than way after or before that time. You also need to avoid giving in to the mid-afternoon dip and having a nap. In the same way that pre-school children who have outgrown their afternoon nap are difficult to settle at night if they do fall asleep in the afternoon, insomnia sufferers who nap during the day are also likely to have more difficulty sleeping that night. It is important to maintain a very regular schedule of sleep and wake times, and naps are completely banned.

If you can't get to sleep within about 15 minutes of going to bed, try getting out of bed and even out of the bedroom and doing something else. When I say something else, I mean something that is not stimulating, such as reading a boring book or just sitting quietly listening to low music. Obviously, if you turn on bright lights and get on the internet or do your laundry, this will be counter-productive. You can return to bed once you're feeling sleepy again. If you don't get to sleep reasonably quickly the second time, then just get out of bed again until you're ready for another try at getting to sleep.

It might seem unnatural to get out of bed when you're trying to get to sleep, but if you lie awake in bed, your body will assume that it is normal to be awake when you are in bed. If you can avoid being in your bed except for short periods of time just before you sleep, you can get your body to associate being in bed with being asleep. This will make it easier for you to get to sleep in the future, as your body will naturally relax whenever you go to bed.

Be consistent with yourself and it will pay off. Remember, you are trying to re-train your brain and the techniques might seem strange, but the research evidence shows that they work. They may not work the first night or the first week, but if you remain consistent, they will work eventually, so be patient with yourself.

ACTIVITY

1. List below some ideas for low stimulus activities that you could engage in if you wake during the night and can't drop back off to sleep.

   _____
   _____
   _____
   _____
   _____
   _____
   _____
   _____

2. Where can you sit outside of the bedroom to wait for yourself to grow sleepy again?

   _____
   _____
   _____
   _____
   _____
   _____
   _____
   _____

3. List your concerns about using the strategies described in this chapter. The next chapter will help you to deal with these.

   _____
   _____
   _____
   _____
   _____
   _____
   _____
   _____

CONCLUSION

Changing behaviors is not easy especially when behaviors have become habits. Nevertheless, nothing will change unless you change your behaviors and although this may seem obvious, putting it into practice is another matter. Take the time and make the effort to address your sleep-related behaviors and you will find that you get results. However, you should not expect that the results will be achieved very quickly. It has probably taken you many months or years to get to the point where you are now with your sleep and it may also take a while to establish a new set of sleep-related behaviors, so please be patient.

REFERENCES

Morgenthaler, T., Kramer, M., Alessi, C., Friedman, L., Boehlecke, B., Brown, T., Coleman, J., Kapur, V., Lee-Chiong, T., Owens, J., Pancer, J. & Swick, T. (2006). Practice parameters for the psychological and behavioral treatment of insomnia: An update. An American Academy of Sleep Medicine Report. *Sleep*, *29* (11), 1415-1419.

Schutte-Rodin, S., Broch, L., Buysse, D., Dorsey, C. & Sateia, M. (2008). Clinical guideline for the evaluation and management of chronic insomnia in adults. *Journal of Clinical Sleep Medicine*, *4* (5), 487-504.

Chapter 9

CHANGING YOUR THINKING

A ruffled mind makes a restless pillow.

- Charlotte Brontë

INTRODUCTION

In this chapter, I will outline how you can change your thinking so that it promotes sleep, instead of undermining it. With the capacity for complex thinking, humans are the only animals on the planet who suffer from insomnia and this is precisely because of our ability to think and drive our behavior as a result of our thinking. You will learn some effective strategies for working on your thinking and also for reducing worry generally. These skills, along with those that you learned about in the previous chapter are key to you gaining refreshing and satisfying sleep. In time and with practice, this will become almost effortless for you and you will wonder how it was ever a problem for you.

WHAT KIND OF THINKING IS PROBLEMATIC FOR SLEEP?

Sleeping is a brain activity and so it is not surprising that your thinking is inextricably linked with how well you sleep. Certain kinds of thinking, such as worrying and ruminating can really interfere with your ability to relax enough to go to sleep or to return to sleep. Thinking that requires a lot of attention and concentration also puts your mind into busy-mode and increases your level of psychological arousal, which again makes it hard to switch off enough to go to sleep.

This kind of thinking includes making calculations, solving problems, doing research or any kind of cognition that requires your brain to be alert and engaged. Similarly, if you are trying to be alert to sounds that your family or neighbors might be making, this hyper-vigilance can intrude on your ability to relax your mind for sleep. New parents, for example, may find it hard to sleep even when the baby is sleeping because they are very conscious of listening out for sounds the baby may make, or they are thinking about the next time the baby may wake and require their attention.

How you think and what you think about is something you can learn to pay attention to and change, so that it is more conducive to sleep; and this is a very important aspect of the CBT-i approach.

SLEEP STATE MISPERCEPTION

> *It was that sort of sleep in which you wake every hour and think to yourself that you have not been sleeping at all; you can remember dreams that are like reflections, daytime thinking slightly warpe*d.
> - Kim Stanley Robinson, Icehenge

It's often hard to tell how many times you wake up during the night, especially if it's only for a minute or two. In general, many of us wake up to ten times per night but we usually have no recall of most of these very short micro-awakenings and they are, for the most part, not a problem for our sleep continuity. Generally, the older a person gets the more they will wake up at night and be aware of those awakenings.

People in their 50s and 60s typically say that on average, they are aware of waking up just under two times per night. People aged 70 and over report waking up just over two times per night. There are certainly lots of people who wake up less or more than two times per night and this is not necessarily abnormal.

Some people are simply more aware of when they wake up, so they may believe that they are not sleeping as well as other people who wake up just as regularly. It's important to remember if you do wake up at night, that you shouldn't get anxious about this happening. Worrying about being awake during the night can just make it harder to get back to sleep.

Sometimes we think we haven't slept at all, when actually we have slept for most of the night. Feeling this way is called *sleep state misperception*. The misperception often arises because a person has woken up numerous times during the night. When combined, these awakenings feel to the person that they have been awake all night. Unfortunately, thinking that we haven't slept at all makes us more stressed about sleep, and this stress in turn can lead to poorer sleep.

PARADOXICAL INTENTION

Paradoxical intention is a kind of cognitive therapy that involves being trained to confront your worst fears about what might happen if you don't sleep, or don't sleep well. You are challenged to try to remain passively awake and avoid any efforts to fall asleep for as long as possible. This therapy is based on a type of learning called *operant conditioning* and the idea that people with insomnia sometimes develop a kind of performance anxiety when it comes to sleeping.

Surprisingly, people who try to do this often experience the opposite of what you might expect and they find that they fall asleep despite themselves. It is thought that this might occur because the fear of not sleeping actually drives anxiety and insomnia. By demonstrating that sleep loss and its consequences are not as catastrophic as you may have imagined, you eliminate your fear and performance anxiety relating to sleep. Paradoxical intention has been studied and found to be effective for people who have difficulty falling asleep, but it has not been studied in people who have other types of insomnia.

USING IMAGERY

Drag your thoughts away from your troubles – by the ears, by the heels, or any other way, so you can manage it.
– Mark Twain

Imagery therapy is not unlike the traditional idea of counting sheep. The idea here is that you visualize neutral or pleasant images or scenes while you are trying to relax and go to sleep. There is no convincing clinical research to support the use of imagery for the treatment of insomnia, on its own or in combination with other therapies. However, we do know that relaxation training is effective and some people respond better to relaxation techniques involving imagery better than to other types of relaxation training.

You will find some useful websites and apps in Appendix 1 of this book that will demonstrate a range of relaxation techniques, some of which involve guided imagery. If you find these techniques stimulating rather than relaxing, then you may be better suited to using other types of relaxation such as progressive muscle relaxation.

COGNITIVE STRATEGIES

Don't fight with the pillow, but lay down your head; and kick every worriment out of the bed.
- Edmund Vance Cooke

The aim of cognitive strategies is to target the unhelpful and self-defeating beliefs, thoughts or cognitions that are contributing to your insomnia. Some examples of unhelpful beliefs might include the following:

- I will never be a good sleeper.
- It is more interesting to be an insomniac.
- I am more productive because I don't sleep as much as other people.
- I can't stick at this stimulus control therapy – it isn't going to work, just like everything else I have tried.
- If I don't sleep tonight, I won't be able to function properly tomorrow and that will be disastrous because…
- These strategies are just giving me worse insomnia.
- I never sleep more than three to four hours a night.
- I haven't slept at all for two whole weeks.
- If I don't get eight hours of sleep per night, I can't concentrate at all.

ACTIVITY

Make a list of all the thoughts and beliefs that you have (about sleep, insomnia and the possibility of you getting better sleep) that could potentially be interfering with your ability to focus less, or worry less, about sleep and sleep loss.

_____

_____

_____

_____

_____

_____

_____

_____

_____

_____

_____

_____

THINKING AFFECTS BEHAVIORS AND OUTCOMES

What a lot of people don't realize is that whenever we are in a situation, we are thinking about that situation, however briefly. We tend to think that we felt a certain way or behaved a certain way as a direct result of the situation and don't even consider the influence of what we told ourselves in our head *about* the situation.

An event or situation does not directly cause psychological pain or distress. If this were true every time the event occurred, the same feeling and behavior would follow - all the time - for everyone! So something else besides the situations themselves must influence the feelings, behavior and other consequences.

The way we *think* about events and situations influences our feelings and behaviors, which in turn, influences the outcomes we experience. So for example, if you are having trouble getting off to sleep, and you worry excessively about the tiredness this will cause you the next day, you are likely to get a different result than you would have if you hadn't worried about it.

It is important to firstly be able to work out what your thoughts, feelings and behaviors are. It can be really easy to mix them up, so identifying what each of them are will really help to improve your awareness of what is happening to you. Below are some examples of thoughts, feelings and behaviors.

Thought / belief (head talk, self talk)	Feelings / emotions	Behavior that results
"I must get at least 7 hours of sleep tonight or I will be unable to present well at that meeting tomorrow."	Anxious	Finding a way to avoid the meeting in case your performance is affected
"I can't go another night with poor sleep."	Apprehensive	Taking of sedative medication
"This stimulus control strategy is just going to be like everything else I've tried – it won't work."	Hopeless	Poor adherence to the strategy for too short a period for it to be effective

ABC OF THINKING

Using the ABC model, the situation or incident is called the antecedent or activating event (A). The intervening thought or self-talk is called the belief (B) and the resulting outcome is called the consequence (C).

I like to use a driving example. If you are driving along a highway and someone in another car cuts across your lane (A), you might feel angry (C) as a result. When you examine things a little more closely, you will realize that it was not getting cut off in traffic that made you angry but what you said to yourself about it (B). For example, you may have said, "Hey that maniac could have killed me!" Or "Bad drivers like that shouldn't be allowed on the road."

While these statements could be accurate, they actually don't make you feel better; they lead you to feel angry and threatened. As a result, you might scream at them, honk your horn, pound on your steering wheel, or even tail the other car to communicate your anger. Your blood pressure could go up and you might even arrive at your destination feeling flustered. It could even spoil your day, especially if you end up in a shouting match with the other driver. Even worse, it could wind up in an accident or assault. It has happened!

If we re-wind the situation to when the other car first cut you off, you could try saying something different to yourself so that the incident doesn't bother you as much. It doesn't matter that it may not be true – the important thing is the outcome for you. For example, you could think, "The driver probably didn't see me." Or "Perhaps the driver has a lot on their mind today."

EXAMPLE TO ILLUSTRATE THE ABC MODEL

Three friends, Lauren, Jessica and Mark, were on vacation in the country and walking along a hiking trail when they came across an unfamiliar, unleashed, large dog.

- Lauren is a veterinary nurse who works with domestic pets every day in a local vet surgery.
- Jessica is a medical receptionist, who was once bitten by a dog and remains fearful of all dogs.
- Mark is a lawyer, who lives in a large city and has little experience with dogs, but saw a news report the night before about wolves stalking children in the area.

Apply your knowledge of the ABC model of how thinking can influence feelings and behavior for each of the three friends.

Person	B = Beliefs	C = Consequences		
	Thoughts	Emotions	Physical	Behavior
	What might each person think?	What emotions might each person experience?	How might each person physically feel?	What might each person do?
Lauren				
Jessica				
Mark				

COGNITIVE DISTORTIONS

One of the interesting things about the thinking part of this equation is that we sometimes tend to default to certain kinds of cognitive distortions or automatic thoughts out of habit. This could be because of our upbringing, because we're having a bad day or because we are feeling low or anxious.

Sometimes we can just get in the habit of thinking in these distorted ways in relation to particular situations. For example, you may tend to think of yourself as unlucky, and indeed you may never have won a significant prize, but there may be little evidence that you are any more or less unlucky than a lot of other people when you really weigh it all up.

Consider this situation: A person survives a terrible accident and comes very close to losing their life. However, they are left with a serious injury that takes months to heal. You could say this person was very unlucky. If they had been in a different place at the time, the accident would not have happened.

Or you could say this person was very lucky. They survived and didn't lose their life and their injuries were able to heal. The outcome could have been much worse. Indeed, the person in this situation will probably recover more quickly and strongly if they view themselves as lucky to have survived.

Cognitive distortions are errors in our thinking that usually contribute to negative emotions. We all make these types of errors in our thinking from time to time. However, when you are depressed, stressed or anxious, you may tend to make them more often.

Types of cognitive distortions		
Distortion	**Description**	**Examples**
All or nothing thinking (black & white thinking)	You categorize incidents in terms of extremes e.g. good vs. bad, right vs. wrong, success vs. failure. You do not see the areas of grey.	"I am a total failure." "Nothing ever works for me."
Overgeneralization	You see a single negative event as a never-ending pattern of defeat. You may use global, sweeping statements. Typical words used include *never, always, nobody.*	"This always happens to me." "Nothing ever changes for me."
Mental filter	You focus on a single negative detail and dwell on it exclusively. Worry is usually a process of mental filtering e.g., you wake twice in one night and see the whole night as disastrous.	"I'm a mess." "My night has been a disaster."
Disqualifying the positive	You reject the positive experiences you have, insisting they "don't count". When you experience a positive, you usually attribute it to some outside factor.	"That was a fluke; it was just that one time." "I slept well last night but that won't last for long."

Types of cognitive distortions		
Distortion	**Description**	**Examples**
4Jumping to conclusions	You make negative interpretations even though there is no evidence to support your conclusions. This distortion can lead to the development of self-fulfilling prophecies. Jumping to conclusions includes two categories: a) Fortune telling: Anticipating that things will turn out badly. b) Mind reading: Believing you know what other people are thinking.	"I already know what's going to happen." "It won't work." "It will be a bad night." "He doesn't think I'm trying."
Catastrophizing	You think the worst possible outcome will happen, without any evidence.	"It's going to be the worst night." "It's terrible when this happens." "This is never going to get any better."
Minimizing	You shrink the importance of your personal needs and desires.	"I don't really need to work on resolving my sleep problem. I'm used to not sleeping now."
Should statements	Should statements include "should", "must", "ought to" and "have to". When they are directed at the self, guilt results from "should" statements. When the "should" statements are directed at others, the resulting feelings are anger, frustration and resentment.	"They shouldn't have done that." "I must sleep tonight." "I ought to be able to get control over this."
Labeling	This is an extreme form of overgeneralization. You attach a negative label to yourself or others instead of describing the unwanted behavior.	"He's an idiot." "I'm an insomniac."
Personalization	You see yourself as the cause of situations that you were not necessarily responsible for.	"It is all my fault." "I am weak – that is

(Continued)

Types of cognitive distortions		
Distortion	**Description**	**Examples**
		why I keep staying up late." "I just can't sleep – that's me."

If you can identify what cognitive distortions you have in your thoughts, you can start to challenge those unhelpful thoughts and develop less self-defeating ways of thinking, thus reducing the intensity and likelihood of negative feelings and behavior.

You need to understand how the ABC model works and how cognitive distortions can get in the way of achieving a positive outcome. Then you will be able to work out how your unhelpful thinking might be contributing to your sleep loss.

Now I'd like you to come up with your own example of something that happened to you in the last week (A) where you found yourself getting upset (C) over something that was really fairly minor. This doesn't have to be a sleep-related example, but it could be. Write down what all of the consequences (C) were. For example, you might not just have got upset; you might have said or done something that you wished later you hadn't. Then fill in the thoughts you had or the things that you said to yourself about the situation (B).

Activating event (A)

_____

_____

_____

Belief/s (B)

_____

_____

_____

Consequences (C)

_____

_____

STOP-THINK-GO TECHNIQUE

The purpose of the stop-think-go technique is to reduce emotional discomfort, increase your ability to think realistically about a situation, slow your reactions down slightly, and increase the likelihood that you will take considered action rather than just react. The stop-think-go technique works like this:

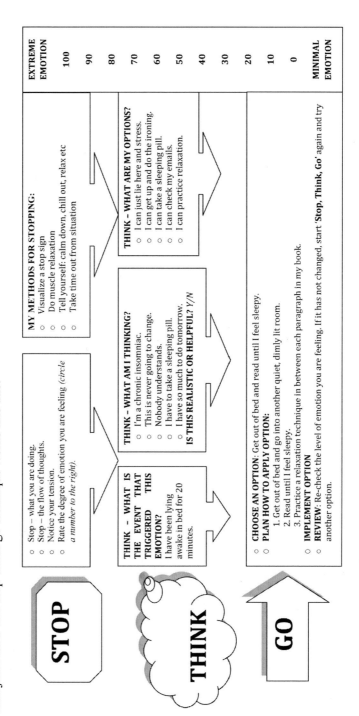

STOP

o Stop – what you are doing.
o Stop – the flow of thoughts.
o Notice your tension.
o Rate the degree of emotion you are feeling (*circle a number to the right*).

MY METHODS FOR STOPPING:
o Visualize a stop sign
o Do muscle relaxation
o Tell yourself: calm down, chill out, relax etc
o Take time out from situation

EXTREME EMOTION
100
90
80
70
60
50
40
30
20
10
0
MINIMAL EMOTION

THINK

THINK – WHAT IS THE EVENT THAT TRIGGERED THIS EMOTION?
I have been lying awake in bed for 20 minutes.

THINK – WHAT AM I THINKING?
o I'm a chronic insomniac.
o This is never going to change.
o Nobody understands.
o I have to take a sleeping pill.
o I have so much to do tomorrow.
IS THIS REALISTIC OR HELPFUL? *Y/N*

THINK – WHAT ARE MY OPTIONS?
o I can just lie here and stress.
o I can get up and do the ironing.
o I can take a sleeping pill.
o I can check my emails.
o I can practice relaxation.

GO

o **CHOOSE AN OPTION:** Get out of bed and read until I feel sleepy.
o **PLAN HOW TO APPLY OPTION:**
  1. Get out of bed and go into another quiet, dimly lit room.
  2. Read until I feel sleepy.
  3. Practice a relaxation technique in between each paragraph in my book.
o **IMPLEMENT OPTION**
o **REVIEW:** Re-check the level of emotion you are feeling. If it has not changed, start '**Stop, Think, Go**' again and try another option.

Stop-Think-Go Practice Activity 1

Okay, now you try using the stop-think-go technique on something that is relevant for you. Use an example of an event that happened to you recently. It does not have to be sleep-related.

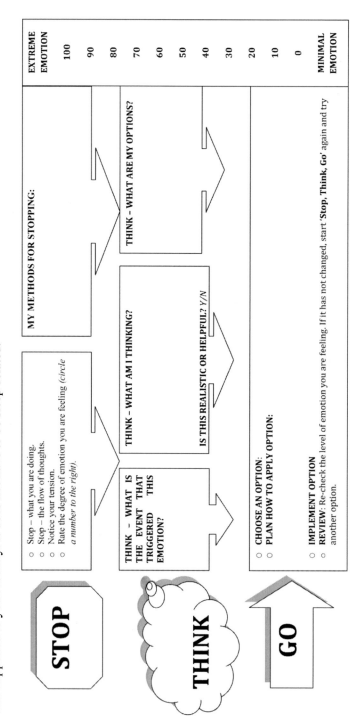

Stop-Think-Go Practice Activity 2

Okay, now you try using the stop-think-go technique on a sleep-related example. If you don't have a recent one, wait until one comes up.

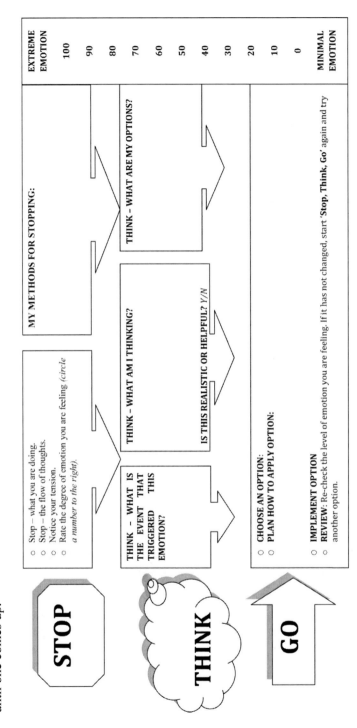

STOP

- Stop – what you are doing.
- Stop – the flow of thoughts.
- Notice your tension.
- Rate the degree of emotion you are feeling *(circle a number to the right)*.

MY METHODS FOR STOPPING:

THINK

THINK – WHAT IS THE EVENT THAT TRIGGERED THIS EMOTION?

THINK – WHAT AM I THINKING?

THINK – WHAT ARE MY OPTIONS?

IS THIS REALISTIC OR HELPFUL? *Y/N*

GO

- CHOOSE AN OPTION:
- PLAN HOW TO APPLY OPTION:
- IMPLEMENT OPTION
- REVIEW: Re-check the level of emotion you are feeling. If it has not changed, start 'Stop, Think, Go' again and try another option.

EXTREME EMOTION	100
	90
	80
	70
	60
	50
	40
	30
	20
	10
	0
MINIMAL EMOTION	

CHALLENGING YOUR THINKING

The result of challenging your original thinking is that you will feel calmer, let it go, and get on with your day without the incident having a major impact on you. There are a couple of different ways that you can challenge your thinking. One is by using the Stop-Think-Go technique. Another way is by using the Rational Disputation technique.

RATIONAL DISPUTATION TECHNIQUE

This technique requires you to dispute the thought or belief that you have in relation to an activating event and then keep a track of what the new consequences are. To start with, you should write some *rational disputations* down, until you get the hang of it and it becomes more automatic.

This step involves challenging or disputing (D) the thoughts or beliefs that you have, so that you get a different outcome or new effect (E) next time. To start with, take the ABC example that you used above and start by brainstorming all the possible things you could have thought or said to yourself at the time that might have been more helpful or less self-defeating. Remember, these challenging statements don't have to be true.

Disputation (D)

_____
_____
_____

The next step is to consider how the outcome might have been different if you had engaged in one or some of these alternative ways of thinking about the situation. This is called the new effect (E).

New effect (E)

_____
_____
_____

WORRY IN GENERAL

We are dying from over thinking. We are slowly killing ourselves by thinking about everything. Think. Think. Think.

– Anthony Hopkins

We know from the research evidence that people who score high on worry inventories are more likely to experience insomnia than people who score low. General worry (not just about sleep but about all kinds of things) can get in the way of good sleep, if you allow it to. Worry is both a cognitive and behavioral response to a current event or even a possible future event (anticipatory worry).

Worry can be used as a way of avoiding the thoughts of feared outcomes and giving a false sense of control over negative situations or possible negative future situations. However, all this does is decrease your ability to work through difficult situations and deal with your underlying emotions. You might not be consciously aware of it, but worry actually contributes to maintaining your anxiety, and thus to maintaining your insomnia. Some key features of worry are listed below:

- It is usually a continuous and nebulous stream of thoughts or ideas.
- It is usually accompanied by feelings of apprehension or anxiety.
- It often concerns potential future events and catastrophes.
- It interferes with the ability to think clearly.
- It can be very difficult to control.
- Everybody worries sometimes.

WORRY ABOUT WORRY

This might seem ridiculous at first, but when worry becomes extreme, as in the case of a person who experiences panic attacks, individuals can become overly concerned about worrying itself. It is not only negative beliefs about worrying that can contribute to maintaining the anxiety cycle. Even positive ideas about worry can be counter-productive. For example:

- Positive: Some people can think that it is a good thing to be a perfectionist, a 'control freak', 'house proud', a 'workaholic' or overly thorough when it isn't really required. They may come to regard worry as a tool that helps them to prepare to deal with possible problems.

These characteristics usually underlie a worrying type approach to controlling things and sooner or later, the worry becomes the problem.

- Negative: Sometimes you might find yourself feeling that worry is uncontrollable or even like you are going crazy or having a breakdown because of stress. This relinquishing of control is just as counterproductive as trying to take complete control.

Prior to identifying these beliefs, it can be useful to recognize the themes of your worrying. This is because avoidance of situations which trigger the worry can also maintain a preoccupation with worry.

Now that we have discussed some of the ways that worry works against you, it is important to recognize how this impacts on aspects of your life. From this you can see where you want to make changes and set yourself some goals.

How does worry impact?	What would the benefits of less worry be?
At work:	
With friends:	
With family or partner:	
With activities you want to enjoy:	
With education or self-improvement:	

WORRY ACTIVITY

Make a list below of all the things that you might be inclined to worry about while lying in bed at night. Some of these things may not be negative. For example, you might need to apply for a visa for a pleasant upcoming vacation. Nevertheless, this could be one of the things that you might think about in bed because it is on your 'to do' list.

_____
_____
_____
_____
_____
_____
_____
_____
_____
_____
_____
_____

Now put this list aside and when you next set aside a special time to brainstorm solutions and prioritize an action list, you can come back to it. Of course, this 'worry time' will be during the daytime or early evening, but not within three hours of bedtime (see strategies for reducing bedtime worry in the coming pages).

WORRY THEMES ACTIVITY

Below is an activity to help you to identify if there are any particular themes to the worry that you might experience. Making a list of your worries can be a useful first step to help you to increase awareness of the areas in your life that you spend a great deal of time and energy focusing on.

Look at the following issue that people commonly worry about and tick those that might apply to you and your worries or add your own:

Health	✓	Social Relationships	✓
Sleeping difficulties		Being rejected by other people	
Poor diet or nutrition		Fear of criticism from others	
Chronic physical problems		Not having close friends	
Digestive problems		Feeling of being left out	
Not exercising enough		Discomfort about conversations	
Other:		Other:	
Finances	✓	**Recreation**	✓
Insufficient funds		Boredom	
Increasing amounts of debt		Uninteresting company	
Unexpected expenses		Too little time for leisure	
Irregular income		Not having enough fun	
Other:		Other:	
Work	✓	**Family**	✓
Unfulfilling work		Worry about family members	
Conflict with co-workers		Sick family member	
Relationship with boss		Relationship with partner	
Wanting a different career		Problems at children's school	
Fear of losing job/unemployment		Lack of a close relationship	
Being rushed or under stress		Problems with parents	
Other:		Other:	
Living Conditions	✓	**Psychological**	✓
Repair and maintenance issues		Worry about worry	
Problematic neighbors		Unhealthy habits	
Unpleasant living conditions		Mental health issues (e.g., depression, anxiety).	
Housework		Lack of motivation	
Other:		Other:	

BEHAVIORS THAT MAINTAIN WORRY

Sometimes the things we do to try to deal with our worries in the short term can actually cause the worrying to continue and worsen. For example:

Avoidance: This involves avoiding situations and people that could potentially trigger worries. By avoiding, you never get the opportunity to prove to yourself that the situation or people were not as threatening as you may have feared. Even if the situation is somewhat threatening as anticipated, you never gain practice at dealing with it and so you don't gain confidence or a sense of competence or efficacy. This usually leads to continued avoidance.

Reassurance seeking: This involves checking with other people that things are going to be okay. It can include contacting friends or family too often to make sure nothing untoward has happened or visiting your physician anytime you experience the slightest change in your bodily sensations. If you engage in a lot of reassurance seeking, you never actually deal with the worry yourself, so it only relieves your worry temporarily. Inevitably, this leads to seeking more and more reassurance from others.

Checking: This involves repeatedly reviewing the things you might worry about, to prevent problems or to ensure that they are in perfect order. This can lead to even greater worry because you may now have additional worry if you don't get to check things thoroughly enough to give you reassurance. Often checking becomes counterproductive as it takes your focus away from the normal range of things you should be paying attention to.

Procrastination: This involves putting off starting tasks rather than risk potential negative outcomes. Procrastination is a form of avoidance and it saps your motivation to address things in your life that need your attention. It also reinforces worry in the same way as other kinds of avoidance.

Suppression of worry: This approach involves trying too hard to control worry, often making it more likely to intrude into your thinking and lead to perpetuation of the worry itself. It works along the same principle as paradoxical attention (see above), but in a way that is unhelpful to you.

What do you tend to do to deal with worry? List below the kinds of things that you do and then identify which of the above approaches fits best with your patterns of dealing with worry. Insight into what you are doing and what you are consciously or unconsciously trying to achieve can help you to be more aware of your habitual approach/es to worry and hopefully, assist you to choose better ways to deal with worry.

_____

_____

_____

_____

_____

_____

_____

STRATEGIES FOR REDUCING BEDTIME WORRY

I've always envied people who sleep easily. Their brains must be cleaner, the floorboards of the skull well swept, all the little monsters closed up in a steamer trunk at the foot of the bed.
                                    David Benioff, City of Thieves

If you tend to worry about general things after you lie down to sleep at night, it is better to set aside a time every afternoon or evening (perhaps before or straight after dinner) when you can think through any worries you might have, and plan any next steps for the following day that will help to set your mind more at ease. Sometimes by systematically thinking through things that worry you, you are able to find ways to better deal or cope with them.

Part of worry is sometimes related to the fear of forgetting some aspect of something you need to figure out. Often by writing these things down, you eliminate the worry that you will forget that you need to address something at some point. Also, this gives you the chance to brainstorm some solutions and get them down on paper for later consideration. You could have a special notebook for this purpose, but please don't keep it in your bedroom!

After you have spent some time thinking through any worrying thoughts, it is good to read a book, watch some TV or listen to some music, in order to take your mind off these concerns and allow you to become more relaxed. The last two to three hours before bedtime should be quarantined for the purpose of getting relaxed and in the mood for sleeping. No worrying or problem-solving should be attempted during this time.

STRATEGIES FOR REDUCING WORRY IN GENERAL

There are three main strategies for reducing general worry. One is to challenge the worrying thoughts, using the ABCDE model outlined above. The other two are problem solving and letting go while accepting uncertainty. If you have difficulty coping with uncertainty, you may actually feel that worrying is useful and engage in it habitually in order to prepare for a range of unlikely eventualities. You may see worry as a way of making life more predictable and preventing unwelcome surprises. You may then be led to believe that worry is helping you to maintain better control.

This is an illusion because worry does not really make you any better prepared and it does not reduce uncertainty. In addition, worrying makes you more stressed and anxious, so you are actually less in control and more emotionally distressed when you worry. Worrying is fairly natural and it can even be helpful if it leads to you taking effective action or engaging in focused problem solving.

You may take action to change the situation or to challenge the way you think about the situation. In other words, healthy worrying can be used a step to adopting a practical approach to prevent a problem from occurring.

For example, I am about to book myself on an international flight. I could worry excessively about the possibility of the plane crashing and this could even spoil my vacation. I could engage in catastrophic thinking about what the experience of a crash would be like and about how my family would have trouble coping without me. Or I could use this worry to look rationally at my travel plans, do a little research into what airlines are the most reputable and check the travel advisory information to ensure that I am not travelling to places that have poor air traffic control procedures in place. Then I could make sure to book flights that I am comfortable with. Having done that, there is no point in worrying anymore because I have done everything in my power to minimize the risk of a plane crash. After that, I could spend my energies on planning a great vacation.

STRATEGIES FOR LETTING GO OF WORRY

Our imaginations can sometimes be our own worst enemies. When you start to worry about something, it is not too difficult to start telling yourself a horror story about what might happen. These stories can capture your imagination and take on a life of their own if you are not careful. One easy technique for managing worry is to notice and briefly attend to a worrying thought and then think about it for what it is, a fiction. You can comment to yourself that you are just doing that worrying thing again. You can even silently laugh to yourself about the horror story you were starting to tell yourself.

Another technique is to think of your mind as a vast, calm, deep lake with small waves and ripples on the surface. The waves and ripples are your worrying thoughts, which ebb and flow and sometimes get slightly turbulent, but then always settle back down on the surface. A similar visualizing technique is to think of worrying thoughts as leaves floating down a gently flowing stream.

Still another strategy is mindfulness meditation. The primary focus of this technique is to focus on your breathing while engaging in calm, non-judging awareness, observing and allowing thoughts and feelings to come and go without getting involved in them. If you notice that your attention gets caught up in the worrying thoughts, just take note of this and bring your attention back to your breathing. Tell yourself that it is perfectly natural for thoughts to arise and for you to pay attention to them, but keep bringing your attention back to your breathing.

The websites and apps in Appendix 1 will take you to these techniques and many others that are useful for becoming more mindful about your thinking and get yourself into a mental space where worries can't take hold or have a great impact on how you feel or function.

CONCLUSION

As a species, humans have been able to gain a lot of benefits from being able to think about our problems and speak about them as well. However, problems do sometimes arise from thinking, especially when we think or worry too much. This really comes into play when it comes to things that we cannot voluntarily control, such as sleeping. As I have shown in this chapter, the only way to deal with this is to think less about sleep and the associated difficulties, to essentially switch off from thinking about it. This element is key to the strategies in this book and none of the rest of it will work effectively if you don't address this aspect. So pay attention to your thinking and when you notice that it is self-defeating, challenge that thinking. You will find that this is useful not just in relation to sleep, but in relation to many aspects of daily life.

Chapter 10

CHANGING YOUR ENVIRONMENT

O bed! O bed! Delicious bed!
That heaven upon earth to the weary head.
                                    - Thomas Hood, Miss Kilmansegg - Her Dream

INTRODUCTION

Now that you know about how to change your thinking and behavior to be more conducive to sleep, there is only one piece of the puzzle left, and that is your sleeping environment. This chapter will detail all of the aspects of your sleeping environment that you need to pay attention to, the most important being light and temperature. Of course, the other important aspect is controlling the amount of stimulation in your bedroom. By this I mean gadgets like television, cell phones, iPads, reading materials, video game consoles and the like. I will discuss why these things don't belong in the bedroom if you are vulnerable to insomnia. Once you have been sleeping normally for several months, you can re-introduce reading materials, but you should remain cautious about anything that requires concentration or attentiveness.

In 2012, the National Sleep Foundation commissioned a market research company to conduct a public opinion poll that involved telephone interviews with 1,500 people between the ages of 25 and 55 (NSF, 2012). This poll invited American adults to respond to questions about key elements of their bedrooms and the effect of the bedroom environment on their sleep. The results of this research showed that respondents tended to rate elements of comfort in their bedroom as having the greatest impact on their sleep, particularly in relation to their mattress, pillows, sheets and bedding, and temperature.

About nine in ten people surveyed in the NSF (2012) poll rated having a comfortable mattress (92%) and/or comfortable pillows (91%) as important in getting a good night's sleep. Temperature also rated highly, with almost seven in ten rating bedroom temperature (69%) as having a large impact on their ability to sleep well. More than half of the respondents rated bedroom darkness (57%) as having a big impact.

LIGHTENED WAKING ENVIRONMENT

As mentioned previously, light is a "zeitgeber" or "time-giver" to the human sleep-wake clock. Morning light resets our circadian clocks each day. Exposure to lots of bright light (especially daylight) will help to keep you awake at the right time of the day: when the sun is up! Letting light into your home environment will assist you in waking up more gently and gradually in the early morning; and ensuring you have light exposure throughout the day will help keep you awake more during the day so you will sleep better at night. This means it will be easier to stop yourself from taking naps too.

It is best to go outside and gain exposure to natural sunlight. Even on an overcast day, sunlight is the best kind of light for re-setting your circadian body clock. However, some people live in locations that are so far North or South on the globe that there is very little daylight in the mornings and afternoons in the wintertime. This can have an impact on sleep patterns in some people and it can also lead to a disorder called Seasonal Affective Disorder (SAD), a type of depression that comes on in the winter months.

If you don't have ready access to natural sunlight in the morning, you can purchase specialized artificial light boxes. The brightness of the light box must be 10,000 lux, so normal fluorescent light is not enough. Even a 10,000 lux light box is not as effective as going outside when the sun is up, even when the sky is overcast.

Ideally, your exposure to this light should be for at least half an hour, between 6am and 8.30am. Light is especially important if you have a tendency to be a night owl because without re-setting your circadian clock daily, you may naturally drift into a *phase delay sleep pattern*, going to sleep later and later each day.

DARKENED SLEEPING ENVIRONMENT

A darkened room is most conducive to sleep, and if there is a streetlight directly outside of your room, or a light on nearby in the house, this may affect your ability to fall asleep. Before going to bed it is beneficial to close the doors, blinds, and curtains, using heavier curtains in the bedroom if a streetlight is a problem. However, because exposure to natural light in the morning is important for the daily re-setting of your circadian clock, the room should not remain darkened in the daytime.

It is best not to have any unnecessary lights shining in your bedroom at night and this includes LED lighting from electronic devices, chargers and digital alarm clocks. If you must have such things in your bedroom, make sure they are covered so that the light they give off does not penetrate the darkness of the room. You can have a night light in the corridor outside your bedroom to light your way to the bathroom if needed but this should not shine into your bedroom.

ROOM TEMPERATURE

Most people have an individual room temperature preference for sleep. Research has found that hot rooms (above 24°C) are associated with more nighttime awakenings, nightmares, increased body movement, and reduced quality of sleep. Research suggests that a hot sleeping environment leads to more wake time and lighter sleep at night, while awakenings multiply. A fan or air conditioner may help, and a humidifier can provide relief if the drier air causes dry skin or airways.

Cold rooms (below 12°C) can also be uncomfortable and are often associated with unpleasant or highly emotional dreams. Adding blankets or wearing thicker nightwear can assist with keeping you comfortably warm at night. In general, sleep scientists recommend keeping your room slightly cooled. Electric blankets can be useful in warming the bed but should not be left on during sleeping. It is better to have warm bedclothes to maintain warmth through the night. Often one bed partner requires a cooler room temperature than the other. In this case, the bed partner who requires more warmth can wear warmer nighttime attire while the room can still be kept cool for both people.

BODY TEMPERATURE

The temperature of a person's body affects their ability to sleep too. Your body tends to cool down as you go to sleep. Having a warm bath or shower in the 2 hours before (but not right before) bedtime is likely to help you sleep, as the cooling down of your body following the bath or shower will prompt you to feel more tired.

Conversely, exercising too close to your bedtime will heat your body up too much (it takes a long time for your body to cool down sufficiently after exercise) and make it harder to fall asleep. It is very important to get your body temperature right because it is so biologically linked to sleepiness and wakefulness. It is better to be a little too cool than too hot, and it is ideal if you can have fresh air circulating in the bedroom, but not if having the windows open poses a security risk or increases the noise in your sleeping environment.

REDUCE STIMULATION

There has been a lot of research carried out about the effects of having technology like televisions in the bedroom. A survey study of nearly 3,400 Grade 5 students in Alberta, Canada, showed that half of the children had a TV, DVD player or video game console in their bedroom, 21% had a computer and 17% had a cell phone (Chahal, Fung, Kuhle & Veugelers, 2013). Five per cent of students had three or more types of devices in their bedroom. Around 57% of the children reported that they used electronic equipment after they were supposed to be asleep. Over a quarter (27%) of the children engaged in three or more electronic activities after bedtime.

Interestingly, the researchers also found a strong connection between electronic devices in the bedroom and obesity, with children with one device being 1.47 times more likely to be overweight than those with none and those with three devices being 2.57 times as likely to be overweight. Children getting as little as one hour of additional sleep had a significantly decreased chance of being overweight (28%) or obese (30%).

There is no reason to think that these findings would be any different for adults. Electronic devices most certainly distract you from the main purpose of the bedroom, that of sleeping. Of course, sex in the bedroom is fine, as people often feel naturally sleepy after sex anyway because our bodies produce hormones to make us more inclined to sleep. This is especially the case for women.

MATTRESSES AND PILLOWS

According to the NSF's (2012) sleep poll, 93% of Americans rate a comfortable mattress and 91% rate comfortable pillows as being important for good sleep. Furthermore, 86% rated comfortable feel of sheets and bedding as important to their sleep.

Choice of mattress firmness will differ from person to person. If the mattress is too firm, you may find it hard to sleep, particularly if you have arthritis. If the mattress is too soft, you may experience lower back pain because you are not getting the support you need.

The best mattress is somewhere in the middle range. Mattress experts say that too often consumers believe that ultra-firm mattresses are good for them, but research on patients with back pain found this was not true and a more supple, comfortable mattress may lead to better sleep.

These days, mattress manufacture has become a real science! There are special mattresses that do not allow the movement of one sleeper to interrupt the sleep of their bed partner and this is especially useful if one bed partner is a restless sleeper. An excellent bed, supportive mattress and comfortable pillows are a terrific investment, so don't scrimp when it comes to purchasing these items.

Give yourself enough space to sleep. If you share a bed with a partner, make sure it is large enough to give both of you room to move around. Replace an old mattress with a new one, and choose a pillow and mattress that fits you best (soft, firm, thick or thin) and will be comfortable throughout the whole night.

When choosing pillows, find the shape and construction that supports your head and neck and that you find most comfortable. And change your pillows regularly. If you have allergies or asthma, you may also wish to purchase hypo-allergenic covers designed to protect you from possible allergic triggers such as dust mites.

There is no hard and fast time frame regarding when to replace your mattress and it depends on your weight and time spent in bed, but most mattresses seem to have a lifespan of around eight years. One way to tell if your mattress needs replacing is to pay attention to your levels of comfort and sleep quality. If you are waking up feeling sore or stiff, this could be a sign that it is time to get a new mattress. You can also check for sagging areas or permanent depressions in the mattress.

It is also important to keep your mattress and pillows clean. You should use a mattress protector cover and pillow protector covers so that you can easily wash them and the mattress and pillows remain clean underneath. Alternatively, most pillows are now machine washable and if you dry them in the clothes drier, this will also kill any dust mites that have accumulated.

Your sheets and pillow cases should be made of breathable fabric and replaced with clean ones at least once per week. According to the NSF (2012) sleep poll, 62% of people felt that a neat and clean bedroom was important to them feeling comfortable enough to get a good night's sleep.

Pillows are important as they are meant to support your head and neck while sleeping. Pillows should help you to maintain a neutral, aligned position in bed and should not cause you to bend your neck or sleep in an awkward position. If your pillows are 10 years old and the thickness of a newspaper, they probably aren't providing you with adequate neck support! Pillows should be replaced at least every 2 years, more often if you find that they have lost their cushioning comfort. You also need to pay attention to the type of pillow you use. There are many different types available now, with varying shapes, degrees of firmness, filling, covering material, and even scent. Pillows should also be checked to see if they have become limp, lumpy or saggy.

Interestingly, the NSF (2012) poll also found that people who make their beds up in the morning were 19% more likely to report getting good nightly sleep than those who did not make up their beds. Clearly, there is some psychological connection between sleeping well and paying attention to the way a made-up bed appeals to the senses.

NIGHTTIME NOISE

While some sounds at night can be comforting, others only serve to keep us awake. Many people are unable to sleep if they can hear traffic outside, someone snoring, children crying or a dog barking. If these things are a problem for you, it is worth considering moving to a quieter room in the house, using ear plugs, putting on the air conditioning or a fan, or acquiring some heavier curtains.

Sometimes it can be helpful to cover-up unwanted noises by using specific, acceptable sounds or music. Machines are available that produce sounds conducive to sleeping, such as sounds of the ocean. Some people find it easier to sleep if they have the radio un-tuned such that they can hear a steady static sound known as *white noise*.

Noises at levels as low as 40 decibels can keep us awake (Okada & Inaba, 199)0. That means that things like a ticking clock or dripping faucet can disturb your sleep. The absence or presence of a familiar noise can also have a negative effect on your sleep. Studies have found that for city folk, sounds such as traffic noise and emergency vehicle sirens can actually be soothing and perfect quietness can cause uneasiness. Nevertheless, one study found evidence that young adults living in an urban environment were chronically sleep deprived due to traffic noise and that this had a negative impact on their general mood (Carter, 1996).

Research also suggests that intermittent sounds such as a sudden shout from outside, a motor cycle roaring past or an occasional alarm are often more disturbing to your sleep than constant noises that you may become habituated to. I once worked on an island that was inundated in the summer time with migratory shearwaters. The cacophony of these nesting birds throughout the night was almost deafening. No-one who came to the island in the summer could sleep for the first two or three nights but then everyone got used to it. However, there were no cars on the island so the sound of an engine in such a natural setting would most certainly have woken up the inhabitants.

BED PARTNERS

The activities of bed partners rated highly in the NSF (2012) poll in terms of impact on sleep, with nearly half reporting a significant impact on their sleep from their partner snoring (41%) and 27% reporting that partner movement had a big impact on their sleep. According to the National Sleep Foundation's 2005 Sleep in America poll, 67% of respondents reported that their partner snored, 27% said their intimate relationship was affected because they were too sleepy, and 38% said they had problems in their relationship due to their partner's sleep behaviors.

People who are dealing with insomnia often worry about disturbing their bedmate and this is quite unhelpful, so a wider, better mattress may help. It may even be necessary to use separate beds or bedrooms while you are establishing new sleep habits. In addition, if you have a partner who snores or is restless during the night, you may need to think about using earplugs, having a wider bed, separate beds or even separate bedrooms. Of course, it is also important that your partner gets checked out by their physician in case they have a sleep disorder such as sleep apnea or restless leg syndrome.

CHILDREN IN THE BEDROOM

According to the NSF's (2005) poll, children had a lesser impact on sleep than bed partners for most people, with only 28% rating children as having a big impact on sleep. Co-sleeping with children is controversial in the Western world and there are some studies showing a link between bed-sharing with infants and sudden infant death syndrome (SIDS). However, the relationship is complicated and a recent review suggested that the evidence in relation to this relationship is low quality (Das, Sankar, Agarwal & Paul, 2014). The review suggested that more studies are needed in relation to bed sharing, breast feeding, and hazardous circumstances that put babies at risk.

Indeed, Asian countries like Japan and China, though developed, have a lower rate of SIDS than Western countries despite a higher rate of bed sharing (Sankaran, et al., 2000; Kibel & Davies, 2000). McKenna and McDade (2005) have suggested that when these figures are considered, a general recommendation against bed sharing might not be appropriate for developing (including Asian) countries in contrast to developed countries where other known risk factors, such as alcohol, smoking, drug-use and obesity might play greater roles. It has been hypothesized that lifestyle and socioeconomic factors may play a role in these risk factors (Blair, Platt, Smith & Fleming, 2006; Moon, et al., 2011). In some cultures, co-sleeping is associated with reduced infant deaths, while in others it is associated with increased deaths. One Canadian study showed that where breast feeding and forms of co-sleeping co-exist, SIDS incidence is actually reduced (Sankaran, et al., 2000). Similarly, in Hong Kong, where co-sleeping is the norm, the rates of SIDS are among the lowest in the world (Davies, 1985).

Chen and Rogan (2004) contend that there is no convincing published research evidence 'of increased risk to a baby from sharing a bed with a firm mattress with parents who do not smoke and have not consumed alcohol or other drugs providing the bedding is arranged so that it cannot slip over the baby's head, and the baby is not sleeping on a pillow, or under an adult duvet'.

It is beyond the scope of this chapter to fully explore the pros and cons of sharing beds with children but it is important to remember that decisions about co-sleeping are greatly influenced by culture. In many parts of the world, co-sleeping with children is the norm, not the exception as it is in countries like the US, Britain and Australia.

The important thing here in relation to sleep loss is considering what is best for both parents and children in respect to getting good quality sleep. Sometimes it is less disruptive to parental sleep to allow children in the parental bed. However, sometimes in the long term, this may not be the case.

PETS IN THE BEDROOM

According to the NSF's (2005) poll, pets had a lesser impact than bed partners for most people, with only 27% of respondents rating pets as having a big impact on sleep. The presence of a pet on the bed can restrict your sleeping space, and is likely to affect your posture. For this reason, it is usually best to keep pets off your bed. If possible, it is even better to keep pets outside of the bedroom when you are sleeping, as their unpredictable activity and noises, can keep you awake. Some pets snore very loudly, make sounds during REM sleep, jump on and off furniture, or patter around on the floor at night. Older pets may even need you to take them to the bathroom during the night, in which case you may have to be creative with solutions such as a pet flap in the door or indoor bathroom mat.

Many people are comforted or feel more secure when their pet is sleeping near them and they find that they sleep better with a pet nearby, so if you would prefer to keep your pet in the bedroom, it will be worth taking the time to teach your pet to use a special pet bed or pet basket placed on the floor and have carpet or rugs in the bedroom so you are less likely to hear them walking about during the night.

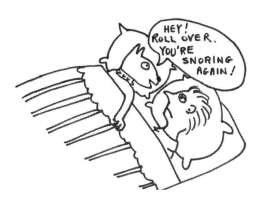

CONCLUSION

There is no doubt that your sleeping environment is something you should pay a lot of attention to in order to provide for yourself the optimal opportunity to sleep well. However, it may not always be possible to completely control your environment and you need to be careful not to get too hung up or obsessed about it. Just as I discussed in the chapter about changing your thinking, you've got to be careful about blaming too much on external causes of your sleep loss. You also need to learn to trust that your body can adjust to almost any situation to meet its drive for sleep. I'm sure you've seen children who seem to be able to sleep through very loud noises and brightly lit shopping centers in their strollers. This is not a skill that is exclusive to children – adults can do it too if necessary. In some sleep deprivation studies, adults have even been able to get sleep while standing up! Nevertheless, if you make your sleeping environment more conducive to sleeping, then it makes sense to do so.

REFERENCES

Blair, P. S., Platt, M. W., Smith, I. J. & Fleming, P. J. (2006). Sudden Infant Death Syndrome and the time of death: factors associated with night-time and day-time deaths. *International Journal of Epidemiology, 35* (6), 1563-9.

Carter, N.L. (1996). Transportation noise, sleep, and possible after-effects. *Environment International, 22*, 105-116.

Chahal, H., Fung, C., Kuhle, S. & Veugelers, P. J. (2013). Availability and night-time use of electronic entertainment and communication devices are associated with short sleep duration and obesity among Canadian children. *Pediatric Obesity, 8*, 42-51.

Chen A, Rogan W. (2004). Breastfeeding and the risk of post-neonatal death in the United States. *Pediatrics, 113*, E435–E439

Das, R. R., Sankar, M. J., Agarwal, R. & Paul, V. K. (2014). Is "Bed Sharing" Beneficial and Safe during Infancy? A Systematic Review. *International Journal of Pediatrics, Volume 2014*, Article ID 468538, 16 pages. http://dx.doi.org/10.1155/2014/468538.

Davies, D. P. (1985). Cot death in Hong Kong: a rare problem? *Lancet, 2*, 1346–1348.

Kibel, M. A.; Davies, M. F. Should the infant sleep in mother's bed? In: *Sixth SIDS International Meeting*. Auckland, New Zealand. February 8-11, 2000.

McKenna, J. J. &McDade, T. (2005), Why babies should never sleep alone: A review of the co-sleeping controversy in relation to SIDS, bedsharing and breast feeding. *Pediatric Respiratory Reviews*, *6* (2), 134 -152.

Moon, R, Y., Darnall, R. A., Goodstein, M. H., et al. (2011). SIDS and other sleep-related infant deaths: expansion of recommendations for a safe infant sleeping environment, *Pediatrics*, *128* (5), 1030–1039.

National Sleep Foundation. (2005). *Sleep in America poll*. Washington, DC: National Sleep Foundation.

National Sleep Foundation. (2012). *Bedroom poll*. Washington, DC: National Sleep Foundation.

Okada, A. & Inaba, R. (1990). Comparative study of the effects of infrasound and low-frequency sound with those of audible sound on sleep. *Environment International*, *16*, 483-490.

Sankaran, A. H., Koravangattu, P., Dhananjayan, A., et al. (2000). Sudden infant death syndrome (SIDS) and infant care practices in Saskatchewan Canada. In: *Sixth SIDS International Meeting*. Auckland, New Zealand, February 8-11, 2000.

Chapter 11

MAINTAINING LONG-TERM HEALTHY SLEEP PATTERNS

Sleep lingers all our lifetime about our eyes, as night hovers all day in the boughs of the fir-tree.

- Ralph Waldo Emerson

INTRODUCTION

Hopefully, you have got to this point in the book and you have been using the approaches outlined in the previous chapters and are starting to see some results. This chapter is a brief one and is just to outline for you what you need to do to maintain the gains that you have made. Changes in behavior and thinking do not automatically stay in place no matter what. Effort is required to bring about and then to maintain change. This effort is yours and yours alone. Of course, effort to maintain change requires commitment, perseverance and discipline.

KNOWING IS NOT DOING!

I must stress here that knowing is not doing. Occasionally, patients who have attended programs that I have facilitated over the years, contact me later and say something like, "Hey, I did your program and it isn't working." Without exception, when I delve a little deeper, I discover that they expected the program to work like a magic wand and they didn't realize (or didn't want to realize) that they needed to not just absorb the information about what to do and what not to do; they also needed to put these things into practice and *use* the strategies they learned about in the program. Intellectual knowledge does not bring about change – you have to *apply* that knowledge and turn that new understanding into action.

You will need to put the strategies that you have learned about in this book into practice on a daily basis and this means that you actually have to be quite disciplined and not allow yourself to slip back into the old habits that led to you sleeping poorly in the first place. This may seem incredibly obvious right now, but habits die hard, and you would be surprised how easily you can repeat the mistakes of the past. Chances are that your insomnia problem was a long time in the making, even if you realized it was a problem quite suddenly. In the same way, healthy sleep will take time to become the new normal for you.

WHAT IF IT HAPPENS AGAIN?

Occasionally, events may happen that result in a relapse of your insomnia. Such events as stressful life situations, work stress, interpersonal problems and travel can suddenly undo some of your good work in overcoming insomnia. In such situations, you may find yourself resorting to sedative medication again. Please do not be discouraged if this happens. You now have the skills and strategies to address the problem and because you have done it before, you will be able to do it again.

It may be easier the next time because you have this knowledge but this will not necessarily be the case. Years may have gone by and age and other factors may contribute to more entrenched sleep problems. Nevertheless, you can still apply all that you have learned in this book, as these strategies can be used by people of any age. You can, and will, overcome insomnia if you are motivated and prepared to work at it using the approaches that have been shown by clinical research to be effective.

CAN I EVER NAP OR READ IN BED AGAIN?

The short answer is yes, but the long answer is that you will need to be careful around reintroducing things that may once have contributed to your sleep loss. When you are completely back in the habit of sleeping well naturally, you may reintroduce something that you used to find relaxing in bed, such as reading. However, I would strongly urge against reintroducing technology, such as television or computers into the bedroom. If you must have a television in the bedroom, do not lie or sit in your bed to watch it, but rather sit in a chair. When you feel sleepy, turn off the TV and go to bed. Try not to let yourself get into the habit of falling asleep while watching television.

Napping is mostly for babies and toddlers, not adults. Some older people nap and that is fine but it shouldn't be from boredom and it should be discontinued if it impacts negatively on nighttime sleep. In general, adults should keep busy and active in the daytime although relaxing activity is also fine.

Perhaps when you are on vacation, you may allow yourself to nap, but even on vacation, you should be careful that you don't get into a habit of totally changing your sleep schedule, so that your circadian clock gets confused. If you have a history of sleep loss or insomnia, you will always have to be careful about sleep scheduling, with a particular emphasis on trying to get up in the morning at roughly the same time each day.

SLEEP IS IMPORTANT

You may recall from Chapter 1 that sleep is important to a wide range of brain and body functions and much of the detail of this remains a deep mystery even to sleep scientists. One thing we do know for sure is that our powerful human drive for sleep shows us that we cannot do without it. Studies have shown that chronic sleep deprivation can raise your risk of health problems such as obesity, diabetes and heart disease and it also impairs your ability to think, react, learn and have a stable mood. Children and adolescents who are sleep deprived are more likely to be moody, impulsive, stressed, unmotivated and to achieve poor grades at school.

The link between sleep loss and obesity is quite a strong one. Research shows that sleep helps regulate the body's production of leptin, a hormone that makes you feel full after a meal as well as ghrelin, a hormone that makes you fell hungry. Sleep loss affects the balance of these hormones so that you feel hungry more often and are therefore likely to eat more and gain weight. Sleep loss can also affect the way your body responds to the release of insulin.

We know that growth hormone is produced during sleep both in children and adults. In children, this is important for growth and development. In adults, it allows for cell repair, healing and recovery from injury and illness. Our immune response is also intimately connected with sleep so that our response to infections is modulated by sleep.

Of course, when you are sleep deprived, you are more prone to making mistakes and having accidents due to lowered levels of alertness. You are also prone to micro sleeps, which can pose risks if you are driving or operating machinery. Unfortunately, motor vehicle accidents that occur as a result of sleepiness are more likely to be fatal than driving accidents from other causes. Although other factors were also involved, human error or fatigue related to sleep loss was linked to some major disasters such as the Chernobyl nuclear power plant explosion, the Three Mile Island nuclear accident, the Challenger space shuttle explosion, the Exxon Valdez oil spill and the crash of American Airlines Flight 1420 in 1999.

Clearly, there are many strong reasons to pay attention to achieving and maintaining good quality, adequate sleep and it should be a priority in our lives. Too often, sleep gets relegated to low priority status compared to things like finishing a job or watching the end of a television program.

If you are reading this book, I presume that you have suffered from sleep loss and perhaps this will make you value sleep more than before and hopefully, you will be less likely to take sleep for granted in the future. I wish you all the very best in your quest for a good night's (and hopefully many good nights') sleep. Sleep well, my friends.

....and so to bed.

– Samuel Pepys

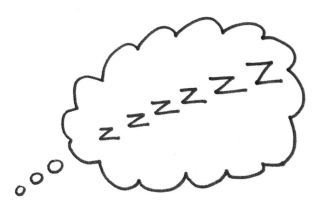

APPENDIX 1. USEFUL WEBSITES & APPS

SLEEP-RELATED WEBSITES

www.sleepfoundation.org

The sleep foundation is a non-profit organization set up to assist people in attaining better sleep.

www.sleepweb.com

This website provides lots of information about sleep disorders and sleep therapies.

http://www.sleepnet.com

This website has a wealth of information about sleep disorders and even includes an online test that you can do to see if you have a sleep disorder.

http://healthysleep.med.harvard.edu/

This website, developed by the Division of Sleep Medicine at Harvard Medical School, focuses on normal, healthy sleep and is a resource from. It has some good video clips about things like taking a behavioral approach to sleep loss and maintaining a consistent wake time.

http://www.sleepforkids.org/

This website is aimed at teaching children about the importance of sleep. It includes games and puzzles that are fun for children to do and that also teach them about sleep.

http://www.bettersleep.org/better-sleep/guide/

This website supported by the mattress industry. It discusses a mattress's life span, explains how to buy a mattress, and compares different types. It also has a link which takes you to a downloadable, eight-page sleep better guide produced by a nonprofit organization.

http://sleepbetter.org/

This website contains loads of information about a range of sleep-related topics.

http://www.wrha.mb.ca/wave/2010/12/cant-sleep.php

This Canadian website contains some interesting reading about people with insomnia and how they overcame it.

SLEEP-RELATED BLOGS

http://scienceblogs.com/clock/2006/06/12/everything-you-always-wanted-t/

This is an interesting and detailed blog about night owls and morning larks.

http://www.letstalksleep.blogspot.com.au/

This blog includes podcasts of interviews with a range of sleep specialist professionals.

http://www.sleep-disorders-gone.com/

This is a blog that has been put together by a recovered insomnia sufferer.

RELAXATION WEBSITES

http://www.beliefnet.com

This website has a great 10 minute video to help you engage in a guided meditation.

http://umm.edu/programs/sleep/patients/relaxation

This website has very detailed explanations about how to engage in a range of relaxation techniques.

http://www.youtube.com/watch?v=-j5Z4E2wkh4

    This is a great YouTube video that will help you learn how to do a breathing relaxation exercise.

http://www.soundsleeping.com

    This website has downloadable music to help you relax at bedtime.

SLEEP-RELATED APPS

    Most of these Apps are free.

Sleep As Android

https://play.google.com/store/apps/details?id=com.urbandroid.sleep
(for Androids)

    The Sleep As Android app helps you track your sleep and shows you graphs of your sleep and the app will also warn you if you have a sleep deficit. The app will record sounds such as when you may be snoring or talking in your sleep, thus potentially alerting you to the possibility that you may have sleep apnea. The app will wake you up gently when you are in light sleep with nature sounds, soothing music or whatever you may choose from the music on your phone or your own special playlist for the purpose.

SleepBot

https://play.google.com/store/apps/details?id=com.lslk.sleepbot&hl=en
(for Androids)
https://itunes.apple.com/us/app/id578829107?mt=8 (for iPhones)

    SleepBot allows you to track your sleep and it also tracks movement overnight, auto-recording so you can hear whether you talk in your sleep, snore or if you're having breathing problems overnight. It also comes with tips to help improve your sleep. It allows you to customize an alarm so that you wake up gently each morning during your lightest sleep phase. You can also listen to soothing ambient soundtracks as you fall asleep. The gradual alarm is based on movements and noise within 30 minutes before the first alarm. It also allows you to graph your sleep length, sleep/wake times, average sleep, sleep debt, and patterns of sleep over time.

Sleep Cycle

https://itunes.apple.com/au/app/sleep-cycle-alarm-clock/id320606217?mt=8 (for iPhones – small cost)

Sleep Cycle uses the iPhone accelerometer to sense your movement as you sleep and involves placing your iPhone under the sheet in the top corner of your bed near your pillow. After five nights of calibration, it collects data on your sleep cycles and patterns and shows you a graph that maps out your sleep for the night. The app even lets you mark conditions for the night on the graphs, including behaviors you may have changed, so you can see their effect on your sleep. A bonus is that it also serves as an alarm clock that tries to wake you when you are in light sleep rather than deep, slow wave sleep or REM sleep. It allows you to set a half hour window for the alarm and also has two snooze modes.

Sleep Time

https://play.google.com/store/apps/details?id=com.azumio.android.sleeptime (for Androids)

The Sleep Time app also involves having your phone in bed with you and uses your phone's accelerometer to detect your movement over the course of the night. It then charts that movement to determine when you entered different sleep stages. You can use it to analyze your sleeping patterns and movements and also as an alarm. The app will wake you when you are in light sleep, so that you don't wake up feeling groggy.

RELAXATION APPS

Most of these Apps are free.

Breathe2Relax

http://itunes.apple.com/us/app/breathe2relax/id425720246?mt=8 (for iPhones)
http://play.google.com/store/apps/details?id=org.t2health.breathe2relax&hl=en
(for Androids)
    This app can be very useful if you feel the onset of an anxiety or panic attack coming on. You can open the app on your smart phone and let the interactive menu guide you through diaphragmatic breathing exercises. Such breathing techniques are known to be useful in managing anxiety, anger and depression.

Calming Music to Simplicity

http://play.google.com/store/apps/details?id=org.t2health.breathe2relax
(for Androids)
    Calming Music to Simplicity is another type of free Android music app that is designed to relieve stress and encourage sleep. This app is inspired by ancient balancing tai chi practices through Chinese music. There are nine selections in all, and the selection chart also allows you to set a timer.

I Can Be Fearless by Human Progress

http://itunes.apple.com/us/app/i-can-be-fearless-relax-remove/id32753817
2?mt=8 (for iPhones)
    Common worries and stress over perceived inadequacies and inabilities can lead to anxiety. This program can assist in helping you to feel less stressed through a series of hypnotic audio recordings.

Nature Sounds Relax and Sleep

http://play.google.com/store/apps/details?id=com.zodinplex.naturesound
(for Androids)
    Nature Sounds Relax and Sleep aims to provide you with the de-stressing benefits of nature sounds. With a wide selection of nature-inspired sounds like waterfalls and ocean waves, this free Android app can be useful in helping you to relax or go to sleep.

Qi Gong Meditation Relaxation

http://play.google.com/store/apps/details?id=com.excelatlife.motivation
(for Androids)

Qi Gong Meditation Relaxation is an Android app that utilizes a series of short videos to unclutter the mind and de-stress the body. Developed by psychologist Dr. Monica Frank, this free app can take your mind off of all the stresses of the world in just a few minutes. With titles like "Mountain Cabin," "Rainbow Emotions," and "Sunrise on the Beach," these videos can be used as a part of other forms of meditation you use to manage anxiety symptoms. Each video is equipped with soothing audio, breathing instructions, and recommendations for muscle relaxation.

Relaxing Sounds of Nature Lite by Red Hammer Software

http://itunes.apple.com/us/app/relaxing-sounds-nature-lite/id345747251? mt=8
(for iPhones)

Relaxing Sounds of Nature Lite brings the soothing sounds of the natural world to your smartphone. This may be useful to you in learning to relax. You can choose from 22 individual sounds, or mix them to create your own nature soundtrack. You can listen to it for a quick way to relieve stress, or to help you fall asleep. This is a free app that works for both iPhones and iPads.

Universal Breathing by Saagara

http://itunes.apple.com/us/app/universal-breathing-pranayama/id4358716
85?mt=8 (for iPhones)

If you're in need for some breathing room, Universal Breathing is a useful app for you. Made for beginners, this app teaches you how to breathe deeply and to retain your breath at intervals for concentrated control. This app is designed to help you with relaxation and anxiety management. Over time, you can perform the exercises for longer periods and potentially gain more effective control over future episodes of anxiety. This app also keeps track of your progress as you move into deeper breathing exercises.

WORRY APP

Worry Box

http://play.google.com/store/apps/details?id=com.excelatlife.worrybox
(for Androids)

The idea of this app is that you place all of your worries in one place outside of your mind, in a "box." The Worry Box Anxiety Self-Help app allows you to create your own virtual box to contain your worries in. This free Android app works similarly to a diary, but it also asks you questions in relation to your own concerns. Questions include whether the worry is controllable and whether it is important. This interactive tool gives you techniques to help you to control anxiety in the long-term. It also helps you let go of current stress. Advice on worry management is also provided.

APPENDIX 2. REFERENCES

Aeschbach, D., Cajochen, C., Landolt, H. & Borbely, A.A. (1996). Homeostatic sleep regulation in habitual short sleepers and long sleepers. *American Journal of Physiology, 270*, R41-53.

Bastien, C. H., Vallieres, A. & Morin, C. M. (2001). Validation of the Insomnia Severity Index as an outcome measure for insomnia research. *Sleep Medicine, 2* (4), 297-307).

Bartlett, D. (2014). Managing insomnia: What we've learnt in the last 10 years. *InPsych: The Bulletin of the Australian Psychological Society, 36* (2), 10-13.

Blair, P. S., Platt, M. W., Smith, I. J. & Fleming, P. J. (2006). Sudden Infant Death Syndrome and the time of death: factors associated with night-time and day-time deaths. *International Journal of Epidemiology, 35* (6), 1563-9.

Carter, N. L. (1996). Transportation noise, sleep, and possible after-effects. *Environment International, 22*, 105-116.

Centers for Disease Control & Prevention (2012). Short sleep duration among workers – United States, 2010. *Morbidity and Mortality Weekly Report, 61* (16), 281-285.

Chahal, H., Fung, C., Kuhle, S. & Veugelers, P. J. (2013). Availability and night-time use of electronic entertainment and communication devices are associated with short sleep duration and obesity among Canadian children. *Pediatric Obesity, 8*, 42-51.

Chapman, D. P., Wheaton, A. G., Perry, G. S., Sturgis, S. L., Strine, T. W. & Croft, J. B. (2012). Household demographics and perceived insufficient sleep among US adults. *Journal of Community Health, 37*, 344-349.

Charles, J., Harrison, C. & Britt, H. (2009). Insomnia. *Australian Family Physician*, *38* (5), 283.

Chen, A. & Rogan, W. (2004). Breastfeeding and the risk of post-neonatal death in the United States. *Pediatrics*, *113*, E435–E439.

Das, R. R., Sankar, M. J., Agarwal, R. & Paul, V. K. (2014). Is "Bed Sharing" Beneficial and Safe during Infancy? A Systematic Review. International Journal of Pediatrics, Volume 2014, Volume 2014, Article ID 468538, 16 pages. http://dx.doi.org/10.1155/2014/468538.

Davies, D. P. (1985). Cot death in Hong Kong: a rare problem? *Lancet*, 2, 1346–1348.

Dauvilliers, Y., Morin, C., Cervena, K., et al. (2005). Family studies in insomnia. *Journal of Psychosomatic Research*, *58*, 271-278.

Drake, C. L., Scofield, H. & Roth, T. (2008). Vulnerability to insomnia: the role of familial aggregation. *Sleep Medicine*, *9*, 297-302.

Groeger, J. A., Zijlstra, F. R. H. & Dijk, D. J. (2004). Sleep quantity, sleep difficulties and their perceived consequences in a representative sample of some 2000 British adults. *Journal of Sleep Research*, *13*, 359-371.

Hublin, C., Kaprio, J., Partinen, M., et al. (1997). Prevalence and genetics of sleepwalking: a population-based twin study. *Neurology*, *48* (1), 177-181.

Karlson, C. W., Gallagher, M. W., Olson, C. A. & Hamilton, N. A. (2013). Insomnia symptoms and well-being: Longitudinal follow-up. *Health Psychology*, *32* (3), 311-319.

Kibel, M. A. & Davies, M. F. Should the infant sleep in mother's bed? In: *Sixth SIDS International Meeting*. Auckland, New Zealand. February 8-11, 2000.

McKenna, J. J. & McDade, T. (2005), Why babies should never sleep alone: A review of the co-sleeping controversy in relation to SIDS, bedsharing and breast feeding, *Pediatric Respiratory Reviews*, *6* (2), 134 -152.

Meddis, R., Pearson, A. J. & Langford, G. (1973). An extreme case of healthy insomnia. *Electroencephalography and Clinical Neurophysiology.*, *2*, 213-214.

Moon, R, Y., Darnall, R. A., Goodstein, M. H., et al. (2011). SIDS and other sleep-related infant deaths: expansion of recommendations for a safe infant sleeping environment, *Pediatrics*, *128* (5), 1030–1039.

Morgenthaler, T., Kramer, M., Alessi, C., Friedman, L., Boehlecke, B., Brown, T., Coleman, J., Kapur, V., Lee-Chiong, T., Owens, J., Pancer, J. & Swick, T. (2006). Practice parameters for the psychological and behavioral treatment of insomnia: An update. An American Academy of Sleep Medicine Report. *Sleep*, *29* (11), 1415-1419.

Morin, C. M., Le Blanc, M., Bélanger, L., Ivers, H., Merette, C. & Savard, J. (2011). Prevalence of insomnia and its treatment in Canada. *Canadian Journal of Psychiatry, 59* (6), 540-548.

Morin, C. M., Le Blanc, M, Daley, M., Gregoire & Merette, C. (2006). Epidemiology of insomnia: prevalence, self-help treatments, consultations, and determinants of help-seeking behaviors. *Sleep Medicine, 7,* 123-130.

National Sleep Foundation. (2005). *Sleep in America poll.* Washington, DC: National Sleep Foundation.

National Sleep Foundation. (2012). *Bedroom poll.* Washington, DC: National Sleep Foundation.

Okada, A. & Inaba, R. (1990). Comparative study of the effects of infrasound and low-frequency sound with those of audible sound on sleep. Environment International, 16, 483-490.

Sankaran, A. H., Koravangattu, P. & Dhananjayan, A., et al. (2000). Sudden infant death syndrome (SIDS) and infant care practices in Saskatchewan Canada. In: *Sixth SIDS International Meeting.* Auckland, New Zealand, February 8-11, 2000.

Schutte-Rodin, S., Broch, L., Buysse, D., Dorsey, C. & Sateia, M. (2008). Clinical guideline for the evaluation and manageemtn of chronic insomnia in adults. *Journal of Clinical Sleep Medicine, 4* (5), 487-504.

Siversten, B., Omvik, S., Pallesen, S., Bjorvatn, B., Havik, O. E., Kvale, G., Nielsen, G. H. & Nordhus, I. H. (2006). Cognitive behavioral therapy vs zopiclone for treatment of chronic primary insomnia in older adults: a randomized controlled trial. *Journal of the American Medical Association, 295* (24), 2851-2858.

Soldatos, C. R., Allaert, F. A., Ohta, T. & Dikeos, D.G. (2005). How do individuals sleep around the world? Results from a single-day survey in ten countries. *Sleep Medicine, 6,* 5-13.

Watson, N. F., Goldberg, J., Arguelles, L. & Buchwald, D. (2006). Genetic and environmental influences on insomnia, daytime sleepiness and obesity in twins. *Sleep, 29,* 645-649.

AUTHOR'S CONTACT INFORMATION

Dr. Sandy Sacre,
Senior Programs Manager,
Adjunct Associate Professor,
Belmont Private Hospital
School of Psychology & Counselling,
Queensland University of Technology
Belmont Private Hospital,
1220 Creek Rd, Carina,
Queensland, Australia, 4152
Tel: 61 7 3398 0260
Email: sandy.sacre@healthecare.com.au

INDEX